DR PENNY SMALL is an accredited practising dietitian and one of Australia's leading nutritionists. She has worked in various local communities encouraging people to make better food and lifestyle choices and with industry partners on improving the nutrition of products on the supermarket shelves. With two daughters and a husband, Penny is a busy working mum whose family has learned to cook through necessity. She currently works with a young dynamic team of dietitians at Nestlé, in Sydney.

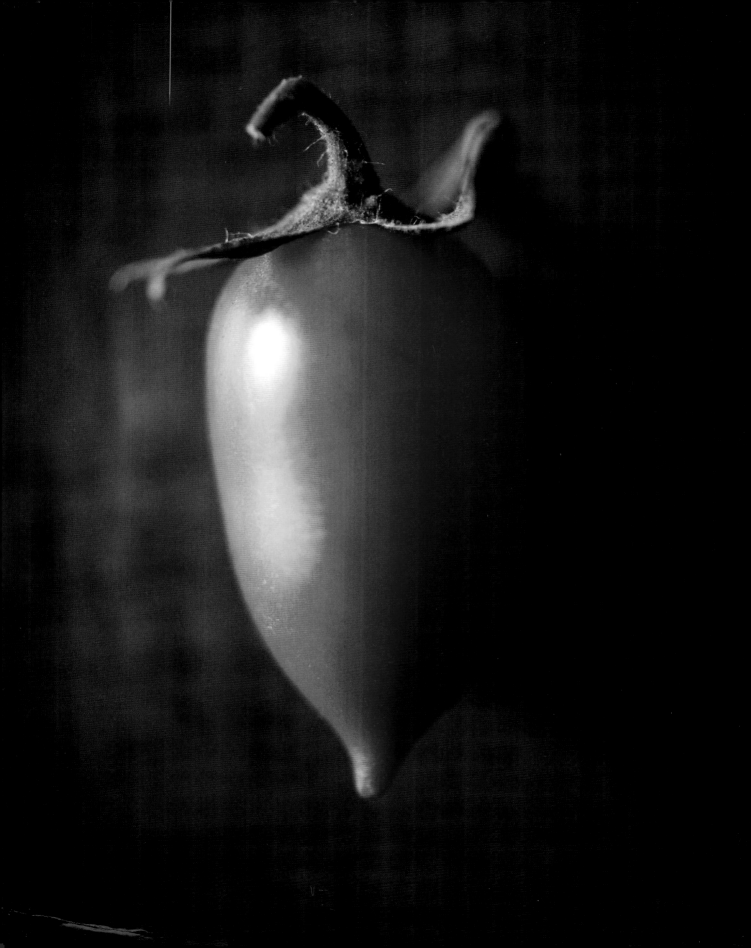

the food lover's diet

Eating your way to a healthy weight

Dr Penny Small

Photography by Adrian Lander

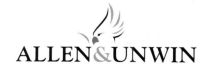

ALLEN&UNWIN

Three recipes in this book have been reproduced with kind permission of Hachette Australia
    from Professor Jennie Brand-Miller's Low GI Diet Cookbook series:
Eggs in Nests from *The Low GI Family Cookbook.*
French Toast with Berry Compote from *The Low GI Diet Cookbook.*
Vietnamese Spring Rolls from *The Low GI Vegetarian Cookbook.*

First published in 2011

Allen & Unwin
83 Alexander Street
Crows Nest NSW 2065
Australia
Phone: (61 2) 8425 0100
Fax: (61 2) 9906 2218
Email: info@allenandunwin.com
Web: www.allenandunwin.com

A cataloguing-in-publication entry is available from
the National Library of Australia
www.trove.nla.gov.au

ISBN 978 1 74237 285 3

Design by Liz Seymour
Photography by Adrian Lander
Styling by Natalie Thomas
Food preparation by Simon Thomas
Project management by Nicola Hartley

Printed and bound in China by Everbest Printing Co.

10 9 8 7 6 5 4 3 2 1

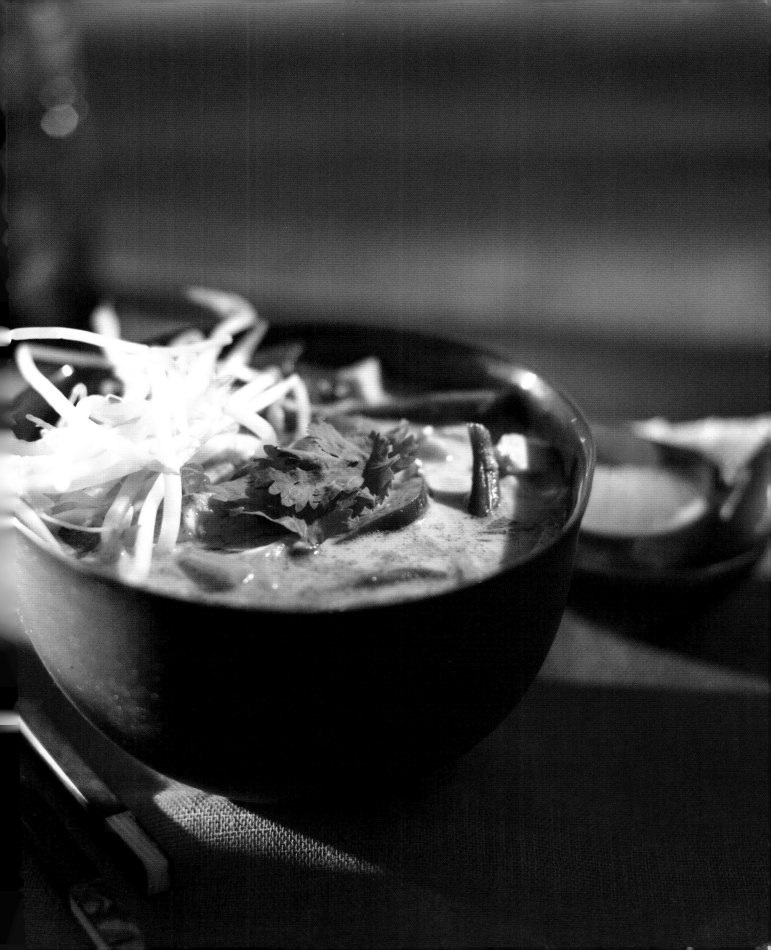

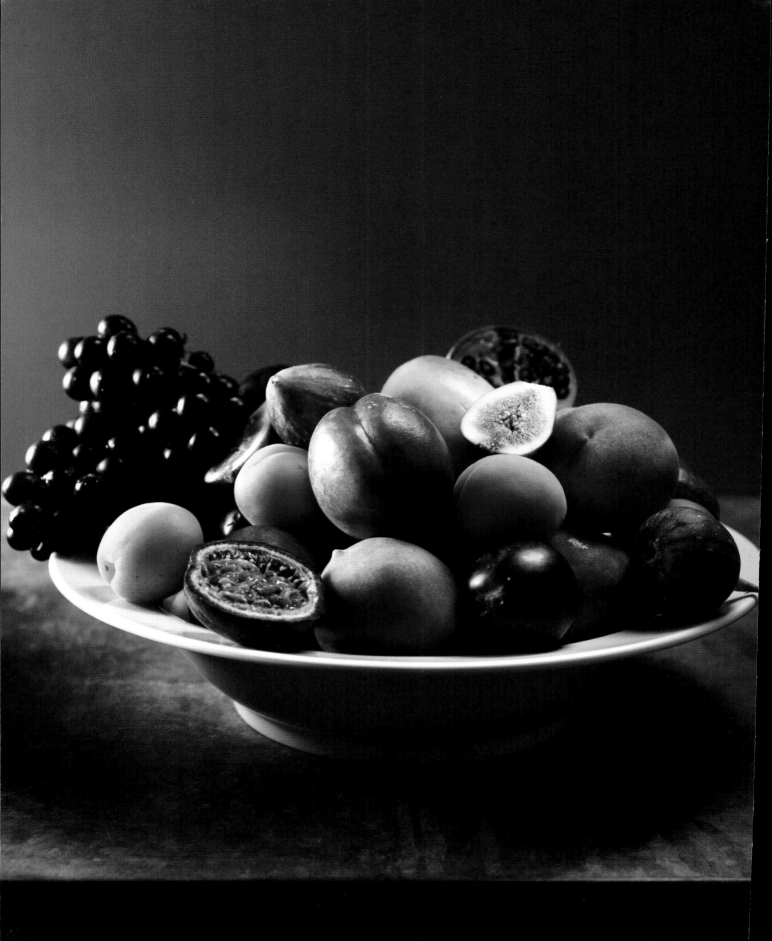

Contents

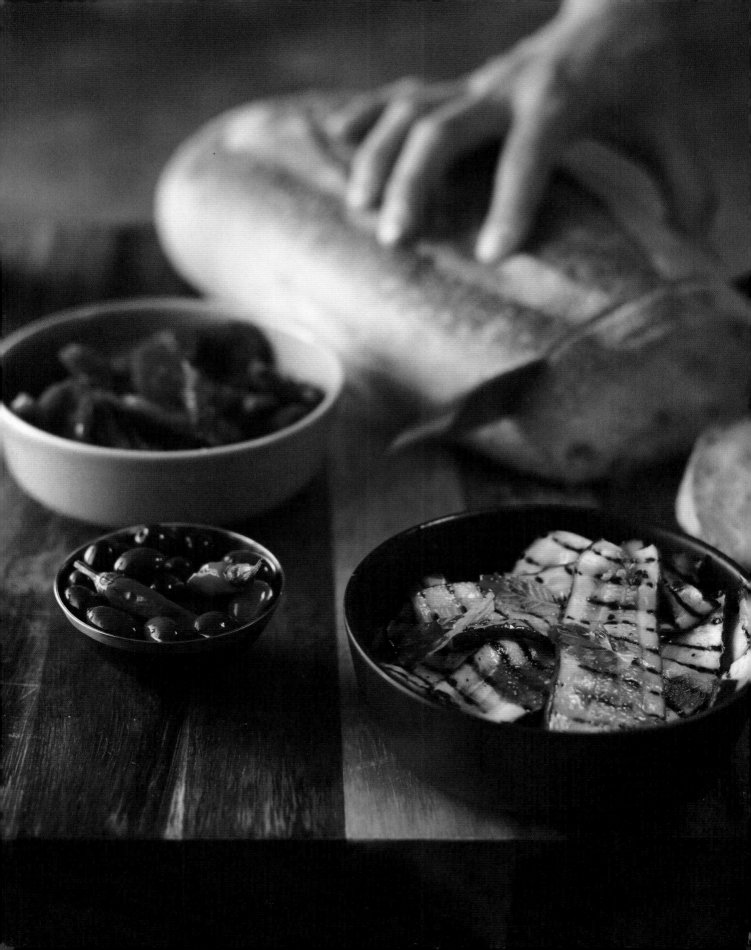

The Food Lover's Diet is a revolutionary do-it-yourself approach for those of us who live in the real world, where food is plentiful, life is hectic and where we can't always get the exercise we need or eat what we should.

Introduction

Food is delicious and nourishing. We have been designed to eat and enjoy food. *The Food Lover's Diet* takes a practical approach to food—it encourages a more intuitive way to eat that includes beautiful nourishing food when we are hungry and allows for treats if we want them. By feeling we are not missing out we can think less about food and get on with life. *The Food Lover's Diet* shows that all foods can have a place in a balanced diet.

This book provides a simple and easy approach to achieve and maintain a healthy weight. It uses a flexible, design-your-own plan that can fit into a sustainable lifestyle and even better, it doesn't leave you feeling hungry, require special meals or keep you tied to the kitchen. It provides tools and strategies that help you see what works well in your life and what could work better. The practical tools include:

- This book, with its simple approach to shopping, cooking and eating and its deliciously effective, family-friendly recipes and ready-reckoner.
- The counter (if you have one), or a notebook and pencil, which enables you to count and track how much you are eating without complicated calculations
- The phone 'app', which lets you download the counts for common foods to your mobile phone.
- The website (www.nestle.com.au) with more recipes, useful tools and nutrition tips.

It's good to remember: Combine 100 counts on your counter or in your notebook with 10,000 steps on your pedometer and achieve your healthy weight goals.

The guidance and tips that follow come from both my own experience and the wisdom of others. I grew up in a family that always celebrated beautiful healthy food and where treats rarely made it to the pantry shelves. As a child I found that it was possible to be overweight on healthy food and came to overdo indulgences

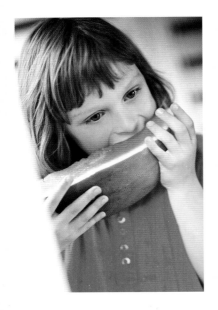

It's good to remember:
The Daily Intake (DI) used in this book are based on adult energy requirements. Although these are different to those recommended for children remember if we are to be role models of good health and teach our families how to eat well, we first have to learn, understand and achieve a healthy way of eating ourselves.

whenever they were around. Yet I observed friends, living in houses brimming with treats that appeared to balance and have a healthy respect for these foods. In attempting to understand why we depend so much on food I became a dietitian. I learnt that if we take a holistic approach to what we eat we can manage food and our weight without depriving ourselves of the things we love. It's about learning to love food and live life in a new way—a way that's good for your body and good for your soul.

Below are a few tricks to help start you on your journey. My hope is that you discover new ways of supporting yourself to achieve your own happy weight—a balance between eating wisely and not going without, and between self acceptance and an eating pattern you can maintain, not just for a week but for a lifetime.

Trick 1: It's about making small changes

Most of us know what we need to do to maintain a healthy weight. Most of us even know what foods to eat. So why can't we do it? Perhaps it's because we think we have to give up the foods we love, or have iron discipline? No, it is simply about building awareness about what we really do and doing it a little differently. Tracking what we eat helps us to do this and make small changes, to do a bit more of some things and less of others.

Trick 2: It's how much you eat that matters

It is less about the foods you eat and more about the serve or PORTION SIZE you choose. It's about moderation. Take small mouthfuls of the foods rich in kilojoules and savour them slowly. Serve bigger portions of the foods lower in kilojoules, making them flavoursome and enjoyable.

Trick 3: It's how often you eat

Achieving a happy weight doesn't mean you have to give up all the foods you love. It's our philosophy that you can eat the foods you like because it is how much and HOW OFTEN you eat them that is important. It's about your everyday food habits. If you frequently include large amounts of rich foods it's harder to find a balance.

Trick 4: Swap this for that

Simple food swaps—substituting better choices for the foods you eat most often, such as choosing lean meats and low-fat milks and yoghurts—will help you achieve your weight and shape goals. And clever swaps can leave room for the treats you love.

Dr Penny Small

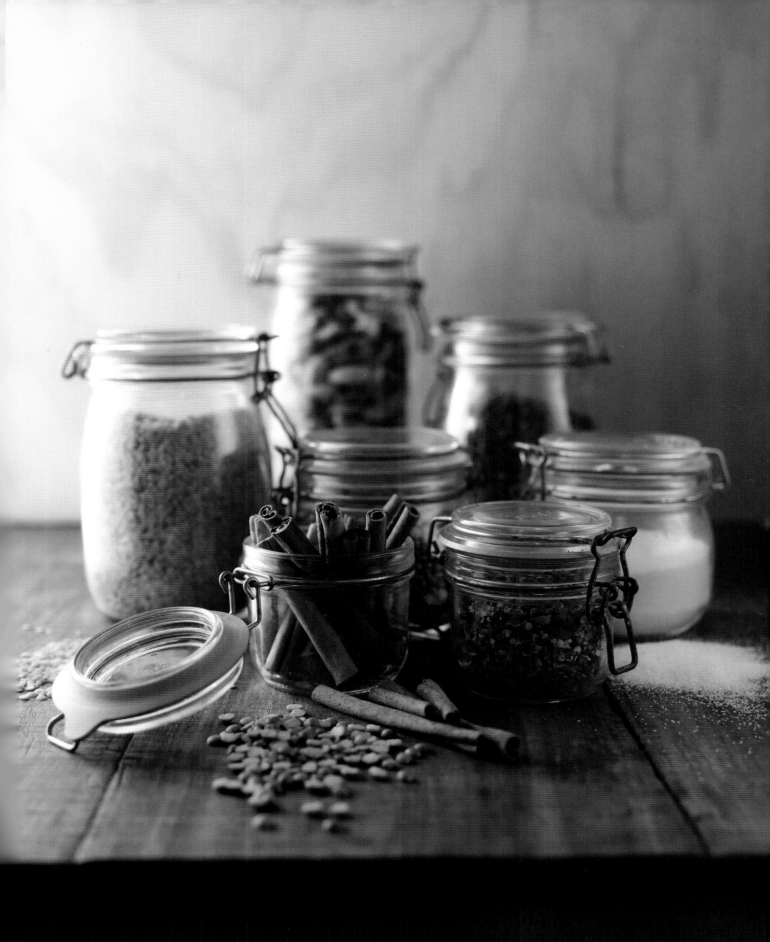

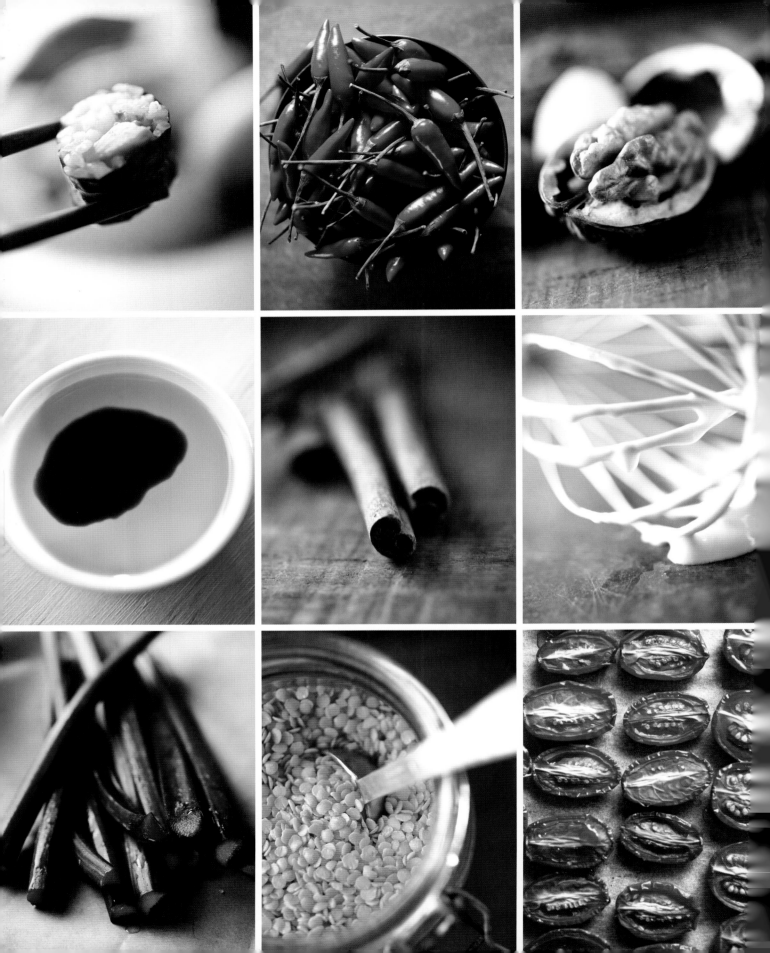

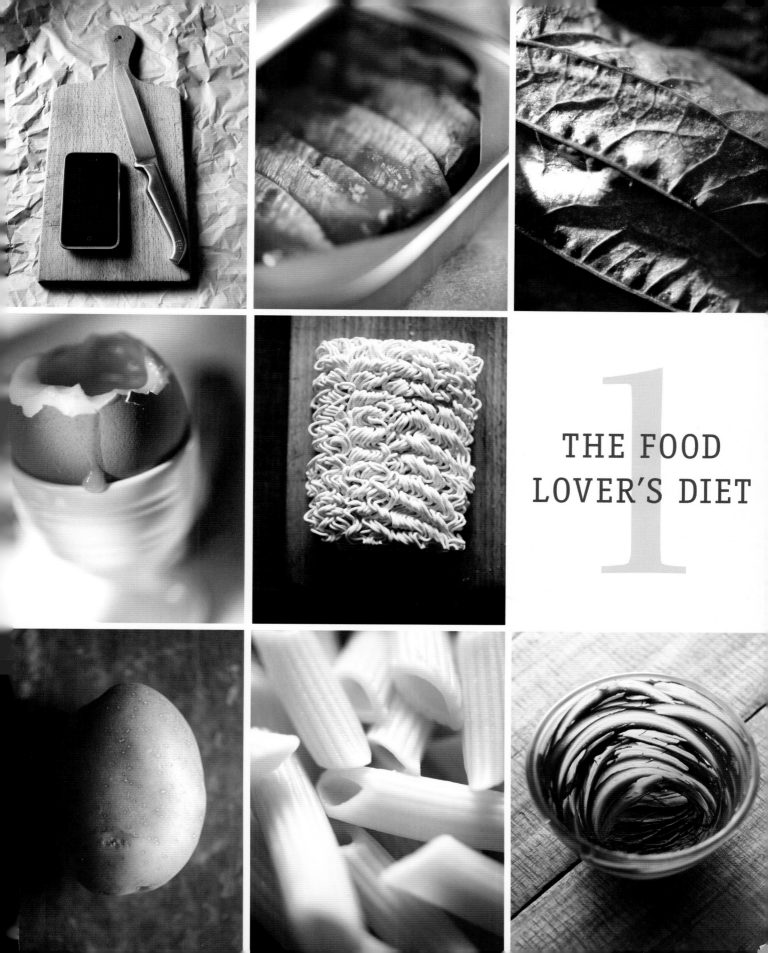

THE FOOD LOVER'S DIET

1

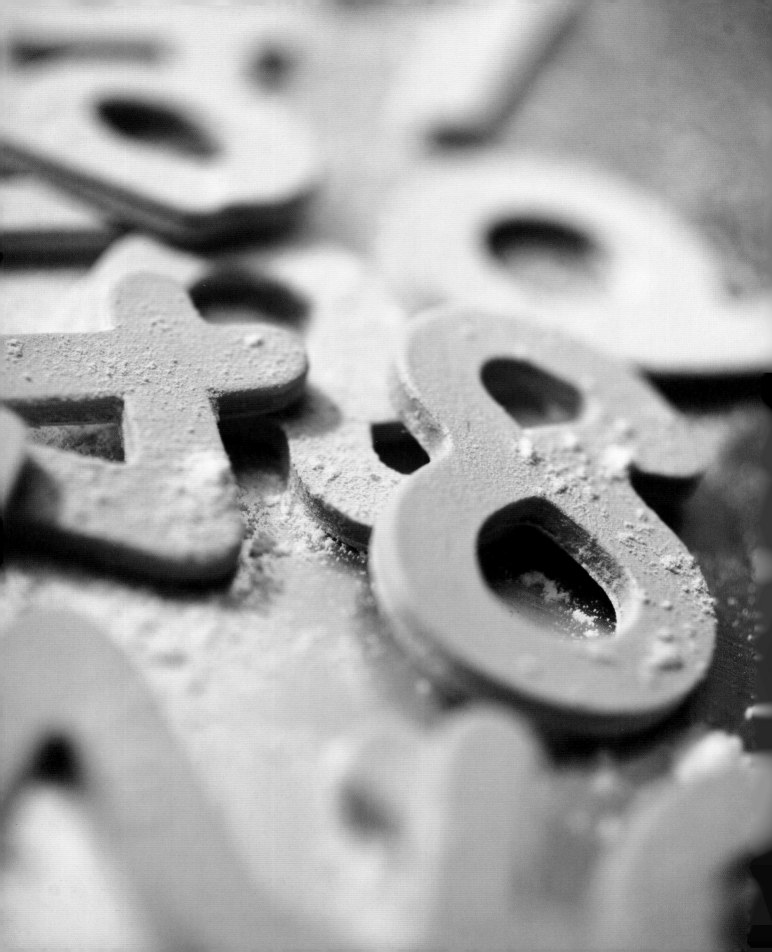

The promise of finally taking control of some of the more difficult parts of life is always exciting, so let's look at how you can do some things a little differently, in a way that enables you to organise and live life your way.

Why count the foods you love?

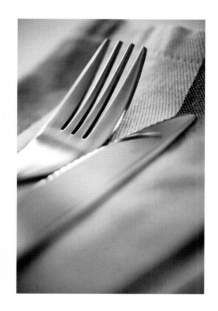

KEY MESSAGES:

- Achieving a happy weight is managing to balance daily energy in and out.

- Energy is measured in kilojoules or calories (the basis for our counts).

- Weight management is all about regulating kilojoules or calories.

Seven things I wish my mother had told me:

1 For a healthy weight, kilojoules in and kilojoules out is what matters.
2 Fat has double the kilojoules of protein or carbohydrate. Water has none. So foods high in fat tend to have more kilojoules and foods high in water tend to have less.
3 Food is to be enjoyed—there's no single food that one needs to feel guilty about eating. What matters is how much you eat and how often. There are many ways to achieve balance, and how you do it is your own choice.
4 Life skills like time management, personal development and taking responsibility have a part to play in all aspects of your life, including your health. Good planning and making good choices help you buy and eat food in a way that enables you to manage your weight.
5 Less is more. Small mouthfuls of food eaten slowly tastes the best and gives the greatest pleasure.
6 Food is one way to cope with the ups and downs of life, but it's not the best way. Seeking out good emotional management techniques that don't include food is a better option.
7 A bad habit is just a behaviour or way of acting that has become routine or ingrained. Learning a new behaviour is like learning any new skill. Every time you *practise* it, it becomes more familiar.

Same **IN** and **OUT** over time
= **weight stays the same**

More **IN** than **OUT** over time
= **weight gain**

Less **IN** than **OUT** over time
= **weight loss**

Good food is the foundation of a happy weight regardless of how much activity we do. Sure, you get to eat more good food if you do more exercise, but in the end achieving a healthy weight is about managing your food intake over and above activity.

For a good weight, exactly *what* food you eat matters less than *how much* because, at the end of the day, it's the *total number* of kilojoules you eat that counts. So achieving a healthy weight is simply about managing your kilojoule intake. Of course, it is important that the kilojoules in the food we eat come with a range of nutrients too, and aren't just energy or 'empty kilojoules'.

To achieve a reasonable weight, we all know we must balance the food we eat with how much our body needs. On one side is **energy in**—what comes in the foods we eat and drink. **Energy**

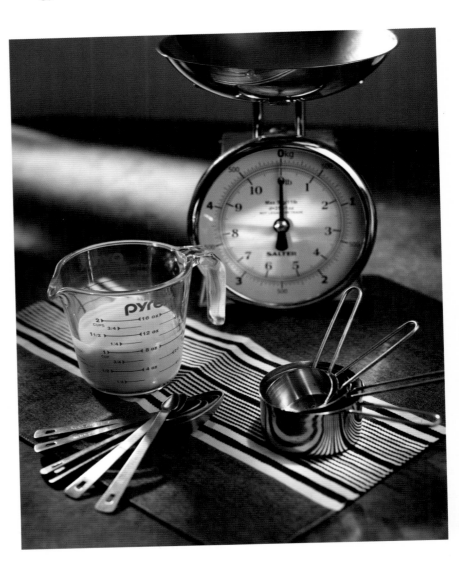

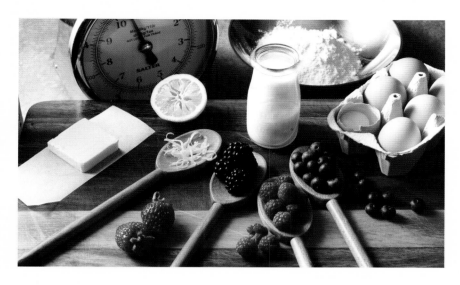

It's good to remember:
ENERGY IN comes from what we eat and drink. ENERGY OUT is what we use up by simply living, breathing, digesting, going to work, exercising and doing our daily chores.

out is how much our body uses to run itself (breathing, digesting our food, etc.) plus how active we are (how much we move).

The amount of energy in the food we eat is measured in kilojoules—a metric measure often abbreviated to kJ. Alternatively, it can be measured in calories—the old imperial measure written as kcal. You will have seen these names on the back of the packaged foods you buy, listed in the nutrition information panel. And, as many of you will know, 1 calorie = 4.2 kilojoules. So, if you want to know how much energy is in the packaged food you eat, check the back of the pack.

When it comes to food, there are three things that determine energy in:

1 The *number* of kilojoules—and our **daily intake (DI)** —in the types of foods and drinks we choose.
2 How *much,* or the **portion or serve size** of those foods and drinks we eat.
3 And how *often,* or **the frequency** with which we choose to eat them.

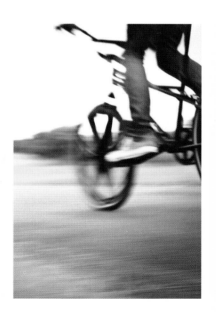

Food energy is important because it is the only source of fuel we have. It fuels the muscles that lift our shopping bags, the beat of our heart, the breathing of our lungs; it feeds our brain and powers all the other amazing body processes that keep us healthy and feeling good. Add to that all the manual activity you undertake in your daily routine—at work, going for a walk, household chores, catching the bus—and you begin to realise how important it is to have a body that is well fed and fuelled, but not over-fuelled and overfed, where our body then struggles to store it.

It's good to remember:
Your ENERGY IN and OUT doesn't have to balance exactly every day. It's the balance over time that determines whether you can maintain a happy weight in the long run.

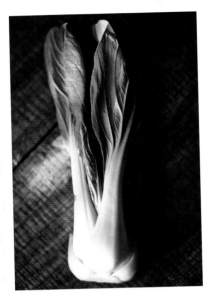

Eating more veggies—stir-fried, roasted, barbecued, quickly microwaved or however you like them—is a simple way of enhancing your sense of wellbeing.

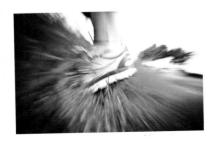

The good news

The good news is that our weight is dynamic and we can change it at any time. To lose weight we need to change our energy balance so the input, or kilojoules eaten, is less than the energy output, or expenditure of living and being active.

For most of us, weight gain comes after periods of time when we did much less exercise or ate far more kilojoules than we needed: holidays, sickness, times of hormonal flux like pregnancy, happy times, sad times, busy times, or whatever. And while we can't undo the past, we can control the future.

Do you remember a time when you or a friend lost weight when being extra busy or very active during a holiday, like when hiking or skiing? It may also have happened unintentionally when you were sick or stressed, or just when choosing to focus more on what you ate or how active you were.

We know weight loss can be achieved—we see people around us do it every day—so we can do it, too. And counting the foods we eat and the exercise we do is the key.

The best news of all is that small, sustainable changes are most likely to last the longest. It's what you do most days and the balance over time that determines whether you can maintain a good weight in the long run.

So, to summarise:

- We can eat all foods, but some foods are best in smaller portions, or eaten less often.
- For those foods we eat frequently, to ensure there is not too much energy going in, we may benefit from making some clever swaps—or choose to have a treat and increase our energy out by going for an extra walk.

There are lots of options to achieve balance in our life, and that's what's important here—you choose what suits you.

To lose weight, you need to change your **energy balance**. It is your choice how you do that.

- Eat fewer foods higher in energy.
- Eat more foods higher in fibre and water content.
- Use the same foods but prepare them differently (less frying, mix with more vegetables).
- Move more, sit less.
- Combine all of the above and do some of everything.

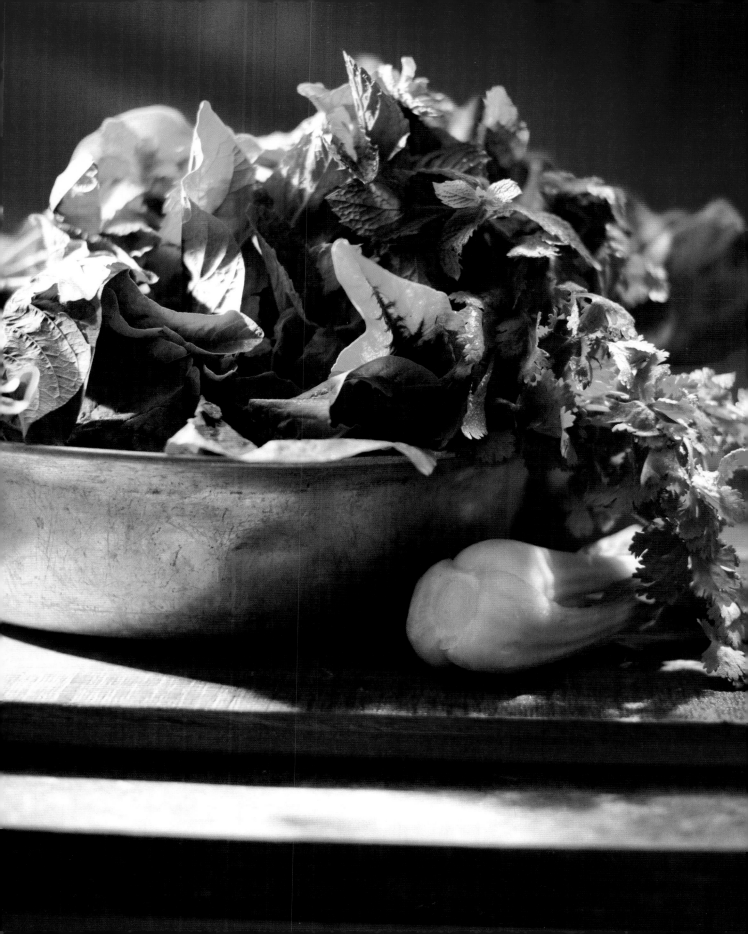

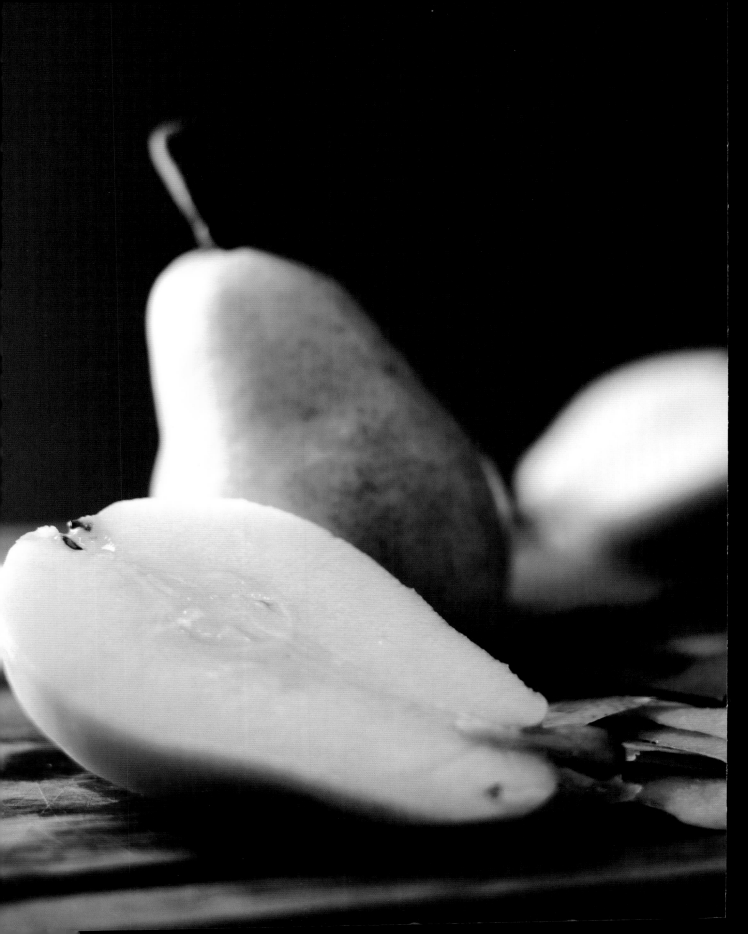

Whether you wish to maintain, lose or gain some weight, tracking and checking what you're *really* eating is a good idea—even if it's just for a short time to get to know more about the foods you're eating.

What is a count?

KEY MESSAGES:

- All you need to know about counts and %DI (percentage daily intake).

- Read the %DI labels and find out more about the food you eat.

- Counts help you make healthy choices—in the supermarket, through the food hall and in the kitchen.

- Keep track of what you eat using the %DI energy labels on food packaging.

- Most of us need around 100 counts a day to achieve and maintain a healthy weight.

If you are trying to achieve a good weight, counting the energy or kilojoules you eat is one way to really help you see how you are doing. By keeping track of the food you eat even for a few days, you learn where the big 'energy in' amounts come from, and you get a sense of what's working well and what's not.

We know that people who track what they eat or keep food diaries are more likely to be successful at maintaining their weight than people who don't. This self-monitoring is a common practice in successful business, too, where the saying is: you can't manage what you don't measure.

The dilemma is that kilojoules are such big, seemingly unmanageable numbers—around 8700kJ a day is the number of kilojoules for a typical active woman or sedentary man—so it makes tracking or adding the kilojoules in the food you eat quite complicated, and you need a calculator to do the maths. To make it simpler, a front of pack labelling system has been introduced on foods called 'daily intake', or DI. And that's what our counts in *The Food Lover's Diet* are based on.

The following may sound a bit complicated, but bear with me as I will be taking you by the hand and showing you how easy it all is in the 'Time to count and track' section (page 16).

The DI package labelling scheme calculates the kilojoules or energy in each serve of the food and helps 'guide' us to eat the right number of kilojoules by showing us what proportion or percentage (%) each serve contributes to our recommended dietary intake—which is just another way of saying 'daily intake'—hence we call it the %DI counts. Now, keeping track of what you eat is literally as easy as finding the %DI count for energy on the front of each pack, then recording or counting these with your counter, on your phone or in your notebook when you eat or cook.

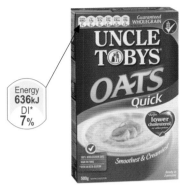

Energy
636kJ
DI*
7%

NUTRITION INFORMATION#

SERVINGS PER PACK: 12	QUANTITY PER 40g SERVING	% DI* PER 40g	QUANTITY PER 40g SERVING WITH ¾ CUP SKIM MILK	% DI* PER 40g SERVING WITH ¾ CUP SKIM MILK	QUANTITY PER 100g
ENERGY	636 kJ	7%	910 kJ	10%	1590 kJ
PROTEIN	5.1 g	10%	12.1 g	24%	12.8 g
FAT, TOTAL	3.5 g	4%	3.7 g	5%	8.8 g
– SATURATED	0.7 g	3%	0.9 g	4%	1.7 g
CARBOHYDRATE	22.7 g	7%	22 g	10%	56.7 g
– SUGARS	0.4 g	< 1%	9.7 g	11%	1.0 g
DIETARY FIBRE	3.9 g	13%	3.9 g	13%	9.7 g
– INSOLUBLE	2.3 g	–	2.3 g	–	5.7 g
– SOLUBLE	1.6 g		1.6 g		4.0 g
SODIUM	< 5 mg	< 1%	100 mg	4%	12 mg

DI = Daily Intake # All specified values are averages.
*Percentage daily intakes are based on an average adult diet of 8700kJ.
Your daily intakes may be higher or lower depending on your energy needs.

ENERGY Use the per 100g column to compare the energy in similar food products. Choose products with the lowest %DI counts (kilojoules).

Tools in the toolkit

Tool 1: Counts are your first tool when choosing foods to achieve and maintain a happy weight. On the front of most packs you will see icons that look like thumbnails. It's the DI for energy (kilojoules) we use here to count. Highlighted in the photo (left) you will see that the DI for a serving of UNCLE TOBYS Oats is 7% or 7 counts. The serving size of the food is stated along side the DI icons.

Packaged foods provide you with a lot of information to help you make informed choices. More information can be found on the back of pack in the nutrition information panel. Look here for additional information on the serving size and %DI may appear again in a column next to the kilojoules. For these oats a serve is 40g. For counts on unpackaged food refer to the ready reckoner in the back of the book.

Tool 2: Something to record your counts. The counter we are talking about is just like other counters you may have seen— to count cricket runs, to count knitting stitches, or even to count sheep. Use the counter to record and add up the total counts of the foods and drinks you consume during the day. If you don't have a counter, a notebook and pencil will do the job just as well. As we said before, if you want to change something, you need to measure it. What matters is that you keep track.

Tool 3: The phone app lets you download the ready-reckoner database to your phone—with the counts for hundreds of foods, including popular brands and basic foods (like milk, meat, fruit and vegetables). The app will inform, calculate, count and do almost everything for you but eat the food itself. Find the instructions on how to download the app onto your phone at www.nestle.com.au

Tool 4: The website www.nestle.com.au has online food diaries to track your counts, tally your daily and weekly intakes, and graph the highs and lows of your week. There are also ideas and recipes, and a community where you can swap stories, provide support and share your successes.

HOW COUNTING GETS YOU BACK ON TRACK

One of my friends, a working mum with a full-time job and a young daughter, was complaining that she really struggles to maintain her weight (and fit into her favourite jeans), even though she is very active most weekends with walks and bike rides with the family. I explained that if you want to change something, you have to measure it first, so we sat down together with a pen and paper to do some counting.

First of all we looked up the number of counts she should have in a day based on her height, age and activity level (the count charts for women and men are on page 25). Her daily count is 98.

We then wrote down what she had eaten the day before, which was a typical working day, and checked the ready-reckoner for the counts in those foods and drinks. (See example following.)

Breakfast = 26 counts
- Two slices thick toast (10 counts) spread generously with margarine (6 counts), one slice topped with Vegemite (0 counts) and the other with half a banana (3 counts) and a heaped teaspoon of honey (3 counts), plus a small glass of OJ (4 counts).

Midmorning snack = 11 counts
- A medium latte with 2 teaspoons of sugar (7 counts), plus one shortbread biscuit (4 counts).

Lunch = 21 counts
- Leftover quarter of a small quiche with salad (14 counts), plus a large bottle of iced tea (7 counts).

Snack = 8 counts
- Two rye crackers (3 counts) with a slice of regular cheese, half on each cracker (4 counts), plus a cup of tea with light milk, no sugar (1 count).

Dinner = 35 counts
- A glass of tonic water (6 counts), a small barbecued chicken drumstick and thigh, skin on (14 counts), a small tub of coleslaw with dressing (6 counts) and a slice of garlic bread (4 counts), plus finishing off her daughter's dessert of ¼ cup custard and ¼ cup canned fruit (5 counts).

Treat = 7 counts
- Two large twists of liquorice (6 counts) and a decaffeinated instant coffee with light milk (1 count).

It's good to remember:
If you want to change something, measure it. Devices that give us feedback, like counters and pedometers, are clever ways of showing us what we are really doing, even for a while to get on track.

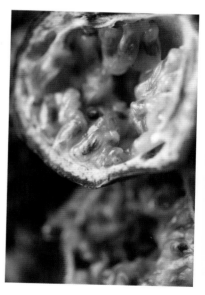

Passionfruit delivers a delicious burst of sweet, tart, juicy flavour, with a small fruit having less than 1 count.

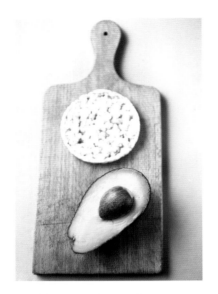

A tablespoon of avocado on your rice cake or cracker is a delicious change from your normal spread but has a similar 2 counts, so remember it makes a similar contribution to your daily energy intake.

Her day's total counts came to 108, so she wasn't too far off her target counts. I explained she had three options—exercising a bit more, eating a bit less, or making some better food and beverage choices. As we looked at the menu we had jotted down, she had a 'light bulb' moment. 'If I just swap drinks like iced tea and tonic water with "diet" versions I will be right on my count target. I'll also try having a "skinny latte" instead of a regular one occasionally.'

When we next met, she was really delighted at how easy the this-for-that approach was for her to keep her counts on target and fit comfortably into her favourite jeans! She also said she thinks twice now before finishing off her daughter's dinner!

Time to count and track

While most of us tend to start a diet at the beginning of a day or new week, in reality we can start at any time. So why not start right now, or next time you find yourself about to eat or drink?

Here's what you do:

- Choose the food (wherever you are—at the supermarket, cooking a recipe at home, or eating out).
- Find the %DI energy count (on the pack, or in the book, or from the ready-reckoner database via your phone app or on the website).
- Record the counts for a serving of this food or drink on your counter or in a notebook (for the first few days it may help to write and click).
- Track the counts over your day, tally them at night and record them in your diary or a notebook.

Tips and tricks

As you get accustomed to counting and tracking, you'll find a few tricks of your own to reduce your counts, such as swapping or substituting. As you start out, here are some of our tricks of the trade to guide you and make 'counting down' simpler. We start with my favourite:

Tip 1: Energy is the ultimate policeman of fat and sugar content

Not all foods were created equal. Fat has twice the counts of carbohydrates (sugar and starch) and protein. Energy in food is determined by the amount of fat (37kJ/gram), protein (17kJ/gram) or carbohydrate (17kJ/gram) present. Alcohol is high in kilojoules, too (29kJ/gram). On the other hand, fibre has very little energy and water has none at all, so now you can understand why high fibre/water foods like vegetables tend to be low in kilojoules.

If you **count** the kilojoules there is less need to worry about the amount of fats or sugars added—the counts automatically account for the fat, sugar and refined starches in foods.

Tip 2: KISS—keep it simple and sensible

Keep the food simple, because when you add extras you add extra counts. For example, if you add extras like butter to vegetables, grated cheese or nuts to savories, sugar or cream to desserts, breakfast cereal or water-based drinks, you add counts because you are adding kilojoules.

A yoghurt or drink that has added sugar and added cream will have more counts than one that is artificially sweetened, plain and/or is low fat, even though the serve or portion size appears the same (like the example on page 18). **So be sensible and keep food simple.**

It's good to remember:
Energy is like the cash register at the end of a big food shop. It tallies up all the kilojoules coming from the sugar, starch, fat and protein contained in the food you choose.

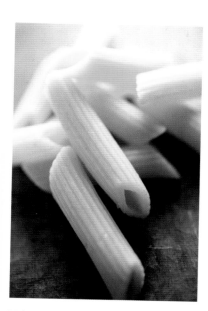

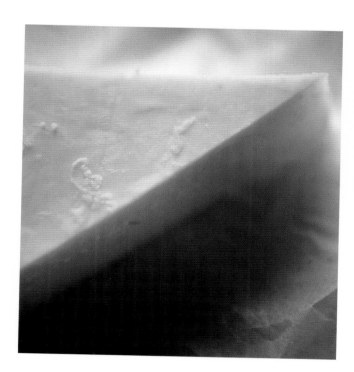

What could be simpler than a small bowl of pasta brought to life with the sharp flavour of freshly grated parmesan cheese. Just remember extra ingredients bring extra counts so only a dash is needed, with 2 tablespoons having 3 counts.

DIET YOGHURT (200G)	LITE YOGHURT (200G)	REDUCED-FAT YOGHURT (200G)	FULL-FAT YOGHURT (200G)
With no added sugar	With added sugars	With added sugars	With added sugars
With skim milk	With skim milk	With reduced-fat milk	With full-fat milk
= 4 counts	= 8 counts	= 10 counts	= 12 counts

It's good to remember:
There's not one food that you can't have, but if you like to celebrate big, celebrate less often.

Tip 3: It's not always WHAT you eat but how MUCH of it

Do you like chocolate? Here is how you can have your chocolate and eat it too—but not the whole block!

Food	Counts
A square of chocolate 5g	1
A row of chocolate 30g	7
A block of chocolate 100g	25
A family block of chocolate 250g	65

Another tip for those who love milk chocolate but can't stop at one piece is to switch to dark chocolate. Dark chocolate is so rich it stops you in your tracks and beats your own worst intentions. The lesson? Stronger flavours can sometimes reduce the amount eaten.

Tip 4: It's not always WHAT you eat but how OFTEN

This tip aims to show you that if you are trying to maintain a good weight, it's what you do every day that counts.

Food counts if eaten every day, versus three times per week or just once a week

- A 50g packet of chips (11) and two cans of beer (7 each) when you get home every night: 25 counts x 7 days = 175.
- A packet of chips and two beers when you're at the pub Friday, Saturday and Sunday nights: 25 counts x 3 days = 75.
- A packet of chips and two beers when you're out celebrating one night per week: 25 counts x 1 day = 25.

The really scary thing about this example is that 175 counts a week if you have that beer and chips every day represents about ½ kilogram extra on the scales.

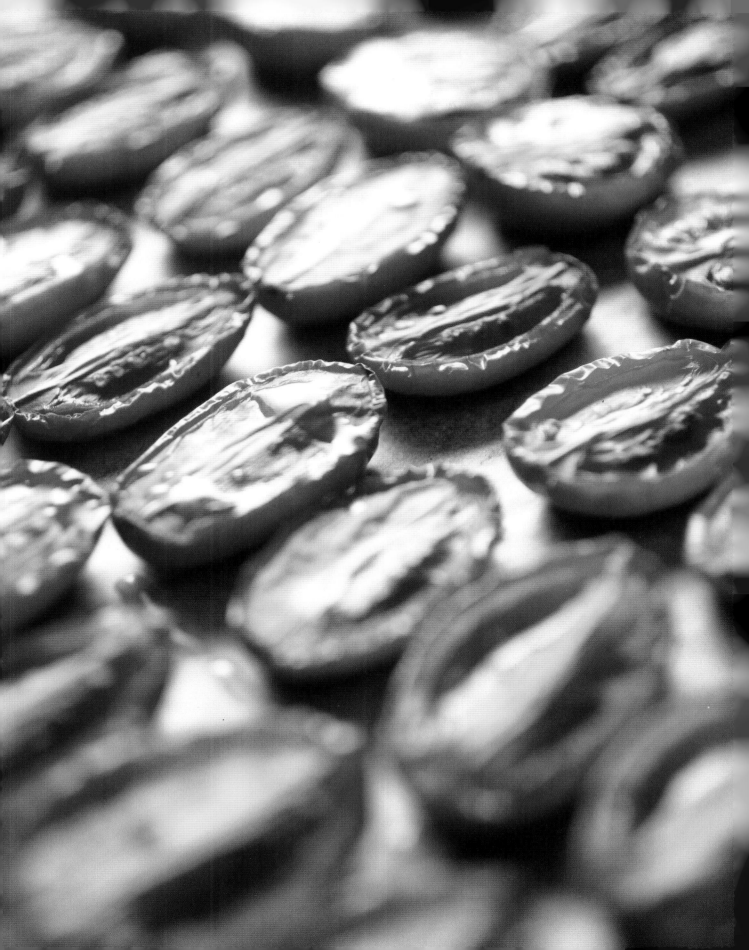

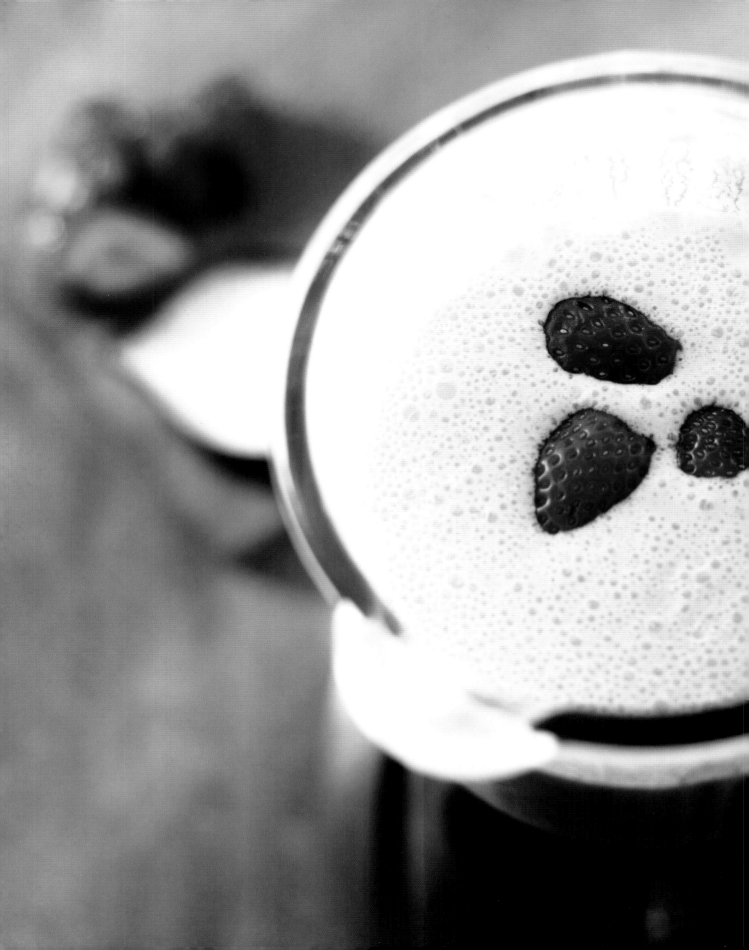

Tip 5: If you like to eat something often, opt for a 'this for that' swap

For some of us it is easier to swap one food for another than it is to give something up altogether. So if something large in counts is featuring large in your life, try and swap down. For example, a supersize drink or juice smoothie may be a great drink as you rush through the shopping mall, but it's also a huge boost to your daily count intake. Simply swapping this for that can really help you to count down. For example, if you swap one 'supersize' banana smoothie (23 counts) for a 600ml diet soft drink (0 counts), you still get the treat, but with a saving of 23 counts per day, or 115 counts and more than ¼ kilogram per week if you're doing it five days a week.

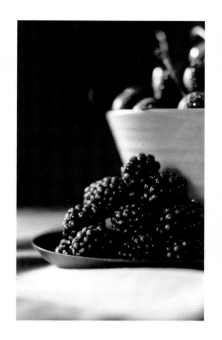

Tip 6: Keeping it all in perspective—it's horses for courses

'Good food bad food' is what all the naysayers would have us believe, but if you substitute better choices for the foods you eat most often, you can leave room for some of the foods you love. Here are two ways of looking at it:

- The 80:20 approach is best if you want a treat daily: Eat most of your food as good, nourishing items spread across the day, and keep the extras and treats as just that … small delicious mouthfuls savoured slowly.
- Categorising foods to *everyday* foods, *sometimes* foods and *occasional* foods is another way to help you balance your food life. If you are having trouble with treats, this may be the best method for you. This involves eating nutritious foods every day, eating the extra foods only sometimes (every few days) and saving the really indulgent treats for special occasions. Remember, treats may be delicious and give you moments of fun or pleasure, but they usually contribute counts with little other nutrition.

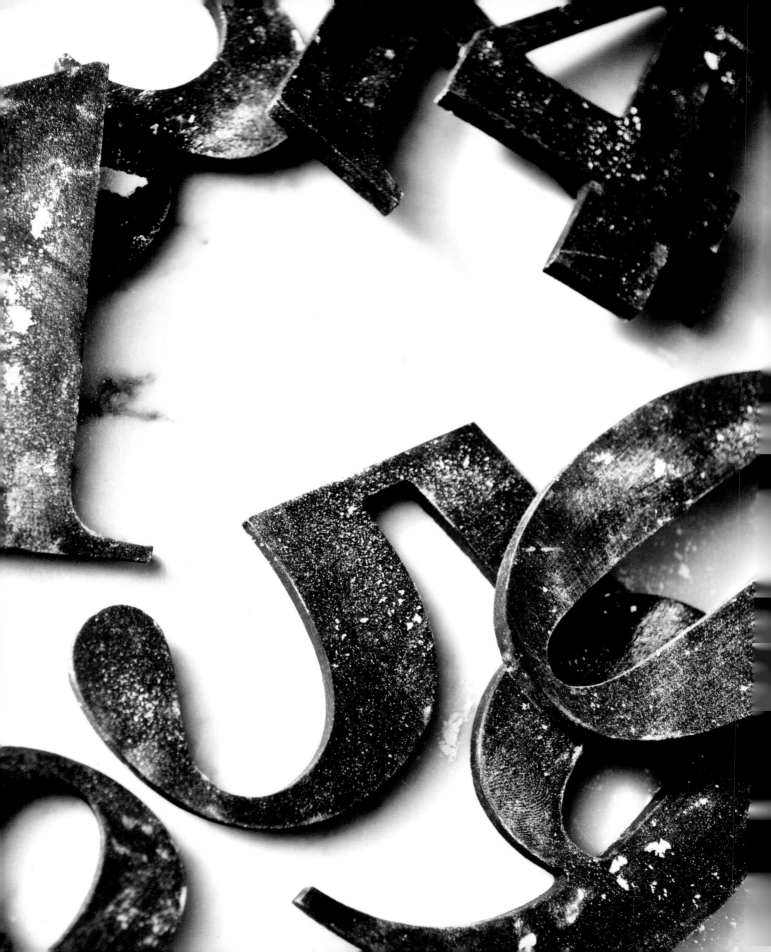

The magic number '100' is a guide to the number of counts a day the average person needs. But we aren't all average. Here's how to calculate how many counts a day *you* need.

How to count the foods you love

KEY MESSAGES:

- Be curious about your eating and drinking habits, and start counting.

- Aim for 10,000 steps and 100 counts a day to maintain a healthy weight long term.

- Remember to try different approaches to find the one that best suits you.

- To lose weight add up your typical daily counts and subtract 25. This and a daily walk may be all you need.

In the previous chapter I explained what a count is and that an average person needs around 100 counts a day (or 100%DI for energy) to maintain a healthy weight. Where does this number come from? It is based on an average Australian or New Zealand adult who is typically a moderately active female or a less active male. If you want to find out more about this, check out the Daily Intake website: www.mydailyintake.net

But since we are all different—what a blessing—many of us have different daily count needs. It's just commonsense that bigger, younger and more active people need more counts than the average person, whereas smaller, older or less active people need less.

How many counts you need a day to achieve and maintain a healthy weight depends on your sex, your age, your height and weight, and how active you are, and you can see the range in our counts charts on page 25.

For example, on my very active days when I have a run, I need 105 counts a day; on my less active days when I am stuck behind my desk or in meetings, I only need 95 counts a day.

Before you make any changes or decisions, it's always good to get the facts straight. Continue to do what you always do, but start counting. Be curious about what you do routinely and when you are out. Do this with an air of investigation and interest—not judgement—this is solely to gain an insight into what you do and the foods you eat. To gain insight into a problem is to half solve it. Do it for a few days, for a week, or however long you like, but just ensure it covers some week days and weekends, both when you are home and when you are out.

Once you keep track of what you are doing, you may find yourself changing a few things. One cannot help but be surprised at what we are really doing.

Grab a pencil and paper now and write down what you ate yesterday, and add the counts. You may find you have a 'light bulb' moment, as my friend did in the example I told you about on page 15.

So now you have the specifics about how many counts you're currently eating. What next?

Choice 1: Keep on doing what you are doing

If your weight is stable and in the healthy weight range, and you and your doctor are happy with it, just keep on doing what you're doing, perhaps making some food substitutions or improvements. Do this in conjunction with a review of your activity level (are you active enough?) and continue to enjoy life with some new found insights into the foods you like to eat.

Choice 2: Work towards bringing your weight closer to the healthy weight range GRADUALLY

You can find out how many counts are for you in the following tables. First, find your age and height on the table opposite, then move your finger through the healthy weight range weights. Next, estimate how active you are on most days of the week by consulting the activity definitions on page 26. Then read along the table to find a prediction of how many counts you need to maintain your ideal weight. For example, a slim 45-year-old woman who is tall (170cm) and slightly active (accounts clerk), is a count 105 person.

Now that you know your counts target, you can plan what it is you want to do. If you are having more counts than suggested and you had a 'light bulb' moment, simply aim to reduce your counts towards your target (somewhere from 80 to 100+) and go straight to the chapter on counting up your activity (page 31). Around 100 counts and 10,000 steps should be all that most of us need to maintain a healthy weight long term.

(If you already eat less counts than predicted in the table or you want to lose weight, don't eat more to increase your counts to reach your target, rather increase your activity or go to choice 3.)

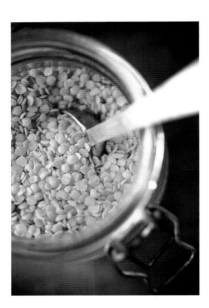

We love lentils; that nutty flavour adds so much to so many dishes. They are high in protein and low in price. What more can you ask for?

Counts estimated for women to maintain a healthy weight

AGE (YRS)	HEIGHT (CM)	HEALTHY WEIGHT RANGE (KG)	NOT ACTIVE COUNTS	SLIGHTLY ACTIVE COUNTS	MODERATELY ACTIVE COUNTS	VERY ACTIVE COUNTS
19–30	150	45–56	82	94	106	117
	160	51–64	89	101	114	128
	170	58–72	97	110	124	138
	180	65–81	103	118	133	148
	190	72–90	111	128	144	160
31–50	150	45–56	84	97	108	120
	160	51–64	87	100	113	125
	170	58–72	92	105	118	131
	180	65–81	95	109	123	137
	190	72–90	100	115	129	144
51–70	150	45–56	79	91	102	113
	160	51–64	84	95	107	120
	170	58–72	87	100	113	123
	180	65–81	92	105	118	131
	190	72–90	97	110	124	138

WOMEN: Bringing your weight closer to the healthy weight range GRADUALLY.

Counts estimated for men to maintain a healthy weight

AGE (YRS)	HEIGHT (CM)	HEALTHY WEIGHT RANGE (KG)	NOT ACTIVE COUNTS	SLIGHTLY ACTIVE COUNTS	MODERATELY ACTIVE COUNTS	VERY ACTIVE COUNTS
19–30	160	51–64	103	118	133	148
	170	58–72	111	126	143	159
	180	65–81	118	136	153	170
	190	72–90	128	145	163	182
	200	80–100	136	155	175	194
31–50	160	51–64	102	117	131	146
	170	58–72	108	123	139	154
	180	65–81	114	130	146	163
	190	72–90	120	137	154	171
	200	80–100	126	145	163	182
51–70	160	51–64	94	107	120	132
	170	58–72	99	113	128	141
	180	65–81	105	120	134	151
	190	72–90	110	128	143	159
	200	80–100	117	134	152	169

MEN: Bringing your weight closer to the healthy weight range GRADUALLY.

* The healthy weight range is considered to be a BMI (Body Mass Index) of between 18.5 and 25 where BMI is your weight (in kg) divided by your height^2 (in metres^2).

Not active = Sedentary lifestyle with no active leisure activities. People who sit and read, work at a computer or desk, or stand still most of the day (e.g., office workers).

Slightly active = Sedentary with some light walking activity but no strenuous leisure activities (e.g., students, drivers, assembly line workers).

Moderately active = Mostly standing or walking during the day (e.g., housekeepers, salespeople, trades people, waiters).

Very active = Heavy occupational daily work or highly active leisure time (e.g., workers in construction, agriculture, etc., high-performance athletes).

Note: If you do sports and strenuous leisure activities (60 minutes, most days of the week) go up to the next activity level.

* Modified from the National Health and Medical Research Council's NRV (Nutrient Reference Values) for Australians.

Choice 3: Using the FAST LANE to achieve a happier weight by reducing your daily counts by 25.

If you don't know what your usual intake is, find your current age and weight in the tables opposite, pick an activity level you know is realistic, then trace across and find the number of counts for you to aim towards. These counts are the regular targets with 25 counts a day removed regardless of your height. This leads to about half a kilo of weight loss a week for most people. If the scales go in the right direction, the tape measure or waistband of your jeans gets a little looser, or you just feel a whole lot better, then you know you are on the right track. If things are not happening as you wish, try a slightly lower count level or increase your exercise commitment and take it from there.

As with any health program, it is always better to do it in conjunction with advice from your doctor or dietitian. An accredited practising dietitian is a wonderful resource if you need some specialist advice tailored just for you. Find a dietitian here:

- Australia: www.daa.asn.au
- New Zealand: www.dietitians.org.nz

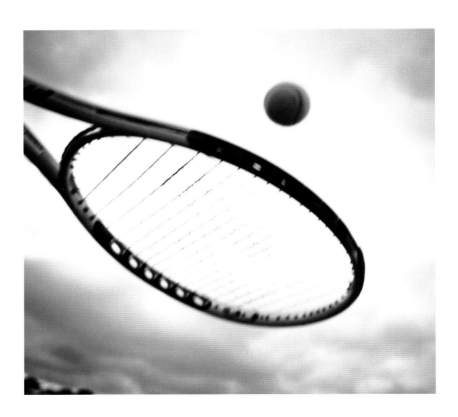

Counts for women in the fast lane

AGE (YRS)	CURRENT WEIGHT (KG)	NOT ACTIVE COUNTS	SLIGHTLY ACTIVE COUNTS	MODERATELY ACTIVE COUNTS
19–30	56-63	64	76	89
	64-70	72	85	99
	71-78	78	93	108
	79-87	86	103	119
	88+	99	116	134
31–50	56-63	62	75	88
	64-70	67	80	93
	71-78	70	84	98
	79-87	75	90	104
	88+	86	102	118
51–70	56-63	59	70	82
	64-70	62	75	88
	71-78	67	80	93
	79-87	72	85	99
	88+	82	97	113

WOMEN: Using the FAST lane to achieve a healthy weight and aiming to lose ½ kilo a week.

Counts for men in the fast lane

AGE (YRS)	CURRENT WEIGHT (KG)	NOT ACTIVE COUNTS	SLIGHTLY ACTIVE COUNTS	MODERATELY ACTIVE COUNTS
19–30	64-70	86	101	118
	71-78	93	111	128
	79-87	103	120	138
	88-96	111	130	150
	97+	120	142	165
31–50	64-70	83	98	114
	71-78	89	105	121
	79-87	95	112	129
	88-96	101	120	138
	97+	114	135	155
51–70	64-70	74	88	103
	71-78	80	95	109
	79-87	85	103	118
	88-96	92	109	127
	97+	104	123	142

MEN: Using the FAST lane to achieve a healthy weight and aiming to lose ½ kilo per week.

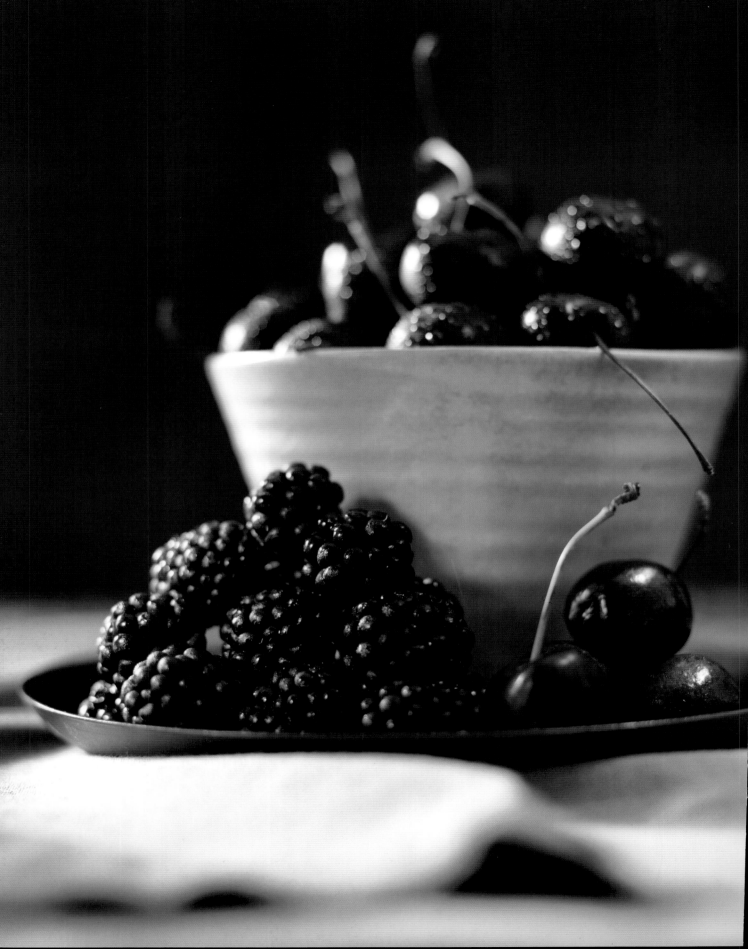

The foods we eat with the nutrients they contain are the building blocks of our bodies. We need to remember it's 'what we eat today that walks and talks tomorrow'. So, if we care about ourselves and our bodies, and we want to look good and feel good, we need to care about what we eat.

Foods that nourish

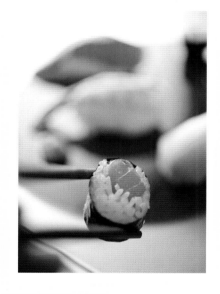

It's the nutrients—the proteins, fats and carbohydrates—that build healthy, energetic bodies, working together with the essential vitamins, minerals and other goodies like antioxidants to maintain these bodies and make them run smoothly. We get these nutrients from eating a variety of fruit, vegetables, wholegrain cereals, legumes, lean meats and low-fat dairy foods.

And if we are clever, we can put these foods into a simple routine of *meals* and *snacks* so we have to worry less about the nutrients and more about enjoying—and we mean really ENJOYING—a wide variety of food. A variety of foods means you get a variety of nutrients, and the benefits of that are incredible.

Establishing a good routine of meals and nutritious snacks helps provide a framework of the key foods that your body needs without you even having to think about it. So, what do we need?

- Foods for growth, maintenance and repair: the protein- and calcium-rich foods that build and strengthen body muscle, bones and teeth.
- Fuel foods for energy and concentration—the carbohydrate-rich, starchy foods and cereals that are slowly digested (low GI), full of wholegrains and rich in the fibre that helps keep us regular and feeling fuller for longer.
- Good fats. Foods rich in unsaturated fats give us essential fatty acids (like omega-6) and fat-soluble vitamins (like Vitamin E). But they are high in counts, so enjoy with care.
- Free foods—the delights of the low-carbohydrate, high-fibre vegetables full of goodness and low in counts.
- Extra foods and treats (sweet or savoury), which we enjoy are optional but can give us a little pleasure that goes a long way.

KEY MESSAGES:

- Focus on feeling good and positive eating; feeling good comes from giving your body what it needs.

- Establish a good food routine with the right counts and your weight will take care of itself.

- If you take on nothing else, remember: variety, balance and moderation.

It's good to remember:
Good food is also about good nutrition—if you don't take care of your body, it can't take care of you.

Here's a simple checklist that helps you focus on the foods your body needs to function at its peak.

YOUR 1, 2, 3 DAILY CHECKLIST FOR LOOKING GOOD AND FEELING GOOD

Eat ONE or more portions of lean meat, fish or other protein-rich food.

Eat TWO portions of fruit.

Eat THREE portions of low-fat dairy or other calcium-rich foods.

Eat FOUR-PLUS portions of cereal and starchy foods, mostly wholegrain.

Eat FIVE or more portions of vegetables, mostly low starch.

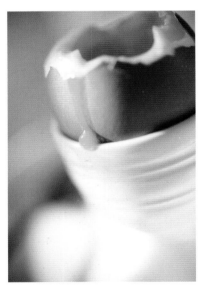

What is more nourishing and nurturing than a softly boiled egg? Versatile, too. Have it on its own or scrambled on crunchy, grainy toast with a twist of freshly ground black pepper.

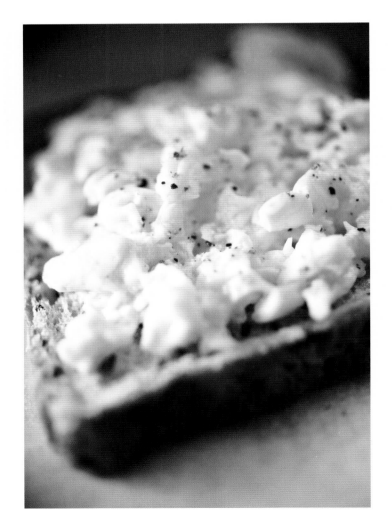

Achieve a happy weight—one step at a time.
Stepping up the pace in your life is simply a matter
of finding activities you like and that fit in with
your lifestyle.

Counting up your activity

KEY MESSAGES:

- Keep track of your activity—a pedometer is the easiest way to do this.

- Set a realistic exercise target you can achieve and maintain and, most importantly, enjoy.

The five simple steps to getting active:

1   Make your plan—succeeding to plan is planning to succeed. This may be as simple as writing out your 'specific' goal: 'I will (walk/swim/jog) each day from (6–7 a.m.)'. Whatever you choose to do, it will probably mean putting out the things you need the night before, or making plans for someone to walk with you, babysit for you, or ask you if you did it.

2   Find your rhythm—plan an activity and a time of day that works for you, bearing in mind your preferences, your schedule and the resources available.

3   Know your motivation—when the alarm goes off at 6 a.m. and you are tempted to roll over and go back to sleep, or a mate gibes you about putting on your sandshoes at lunchtime, it's worth knowing, writing or repeating the reason you are doing this (e.g., 'Each day, in my own way, I am becoming slimmer and fitter').

4   Monitor your progress—a pedometer, a chart to tick off, or tracking your progress on the web (there are lots of great sites) is essential to most people's success. Start off with a three-day commitment and then review your progress.

5   Focus on solutions, not on problems—if your needs or circumstances change, concentrate on finding a new solution to accommodate your activity and don't get stuck in the problem. A 'solution focus' approach allows you to still be 'on the case' and not throw the towel in when life throws up its inevitable barriers. Success comes from knowing you can be flexible and kind to yourself, so leave behind the 'all or nothing' thinking.

Stepping up the pace

One of the joys of working as a dietitian in the community was seeing people come back brimming with vitality after they had started their new health and exercise program. Regular exercise brings oxygen to your skin and your body, and it takes so little time for you to feel energised and glowing with good health.

Amazingly, it brings so many benefits to other parts of your life. And if research has not proved it yet, it looks to me that people who do regular exercise age better, maintaining more flexibility and looking younger. So much return for such little effort.

Regular exercise also:

- Uses up counts and burns kilojoules.
- Reduces stress.
- Tones and slims your body.
- Increases lean body mass (metabolic active muscle tissue).
- Reduces the chance of developing chronic disease such as diabetes and heart disease.
- Helps lower risk factors such as blood pressure, cholesterol and elevated blood glucose.
- Improves mood.
- Improves sleep (if you don't leave your exercise too late in the evening).
- Improves skin and complexion.
- Strengthens your muscles.
- Strengthens your bones (with weight-bearing exercise like walking or pilates).
- Can be free and can be done anywhere at any time.
- Can be whatever you need it to be—fun, social, loud and competitive, or a chance for silence, time out and solitude.

Moderate exercise combined with a few clever food changes is a good strategy to achieve a happy weight.

Becoming a big spender—on counts, that is

The fabulous 'feel good and look younger' benefits of activity also help you maintain a happy weight. Exercise requires food to fuel it, so this means you either:

- Eat more than when you were not exercising and still maintain the same weight.
- Reduce the amount of food you need to cut back on if you are planning to lose weight.
- Lose weight faster if you are already eating less to return to a healthy weight range.

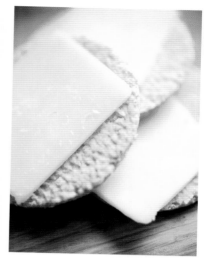

Cheese and bikkies can be a simple satisfying snack when you are on the run.

10,000 STEPS—PEDOMETERS AND COUNTING YOUR WAY TO GOOD HEALTH

The 10,000 Steps program started in the town of Rockhampton, Queensland. The Queensland Government felt significant health and wellbeing benefits could be achieved by encouraging Australians to move more by taking 10,000 steps a day. It was a simple and highly successful plan to help people increase their daily activity with the use of a self-counting pedometer. Pedometers count how many steps you walk, accumulating both the 'incidental' and planned physical activity you undertake as part of your everyday living.

Pedometers come in different shapes and sizes, and with different functions and price points, but most importantly they track your steps each day and help you to increase the number of steps you take over time.

Fit a pedometer on your waistband and walk through a normal day, then aim to increase your daily average by either:

- Adding 500 steps to your daily average each day, or every few days, or as your fitness allows it.
- Adding 2000 steps more each week.

If your fitness and health is already good and you've just been a bit slack lately, aim to do 10,000 steps most days of the week.

Depending on how active you are during a typical day, achieving 10,000 steps for most people means adding a 45–60 minute walk or a half-hour jog. If you really are inactive during the day, an average person can complete the whole 10,000 steps in a 100 minute walking session at a typical pace of 100 steps per minute. It's fun to test yourself and see what your 'step in time' is.

And remember, if you invest in a good quality pedometer, your pedometer's a great self-monitoring tool. It will become your most honest friend, giving you the feedback you need to make a successful behaviour change.

The 10,000 Steps program still continues today, and you can get support, free resources and information online at: www.10000steps.org.au.

To help with your planning, here are some rough guidelines to convert your steps on the pedometer:

- 1 count or 87 kilojoules fuels around 400 steps.
- 1km is around 1250 steps (bigger strider) to 1550 steps (smaller strider).
- 4km walk is around a 50 (bigger strider) to 60 minute walk (smaller strider).
- 1km walking equals around 4km cycling or 1550 steps.
- 1 minute moderate activity is around 100 steps.
- 10 minutes walking is around 1000 steps (800m or 650m).
- 100 minutes (1hr 40min) is around 10,000 steps (8km or 6.5km).

But:

- 1 minute vigorous activity equals around 200 steps ... so 10 minutes jogging or high-intensity sport is around 2000 steps. How come? Because when you run you cover the same distance in half the time and you burn more counts, so even though you really do the same number of steps, they give you a double-bonus step score because it's more intense.

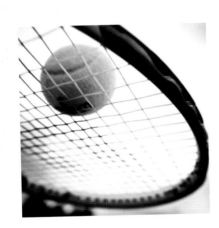

Counting steps is a bit of fun, but remember the terrain, how fast you walk and stride out, your height and your weight will change these figures. Best of all, attach a pedometer and create your own numbers.

A useful way of finding activity to fit into your lifestyle is to think of different ways you can incorporate it into your life and make the most of everyday moves:

- Incidental—walk up to the corner store to get what you need, climb the stairs to see a colleague and ditch the email, or simply fidget a lot!
- Leisure—a game of tennis, a coastal walk, a bike ride, a surf at the beach, a run with the dog.
- Social—a hit of squash, touch footie with the kids in the park, a walk with a friend.

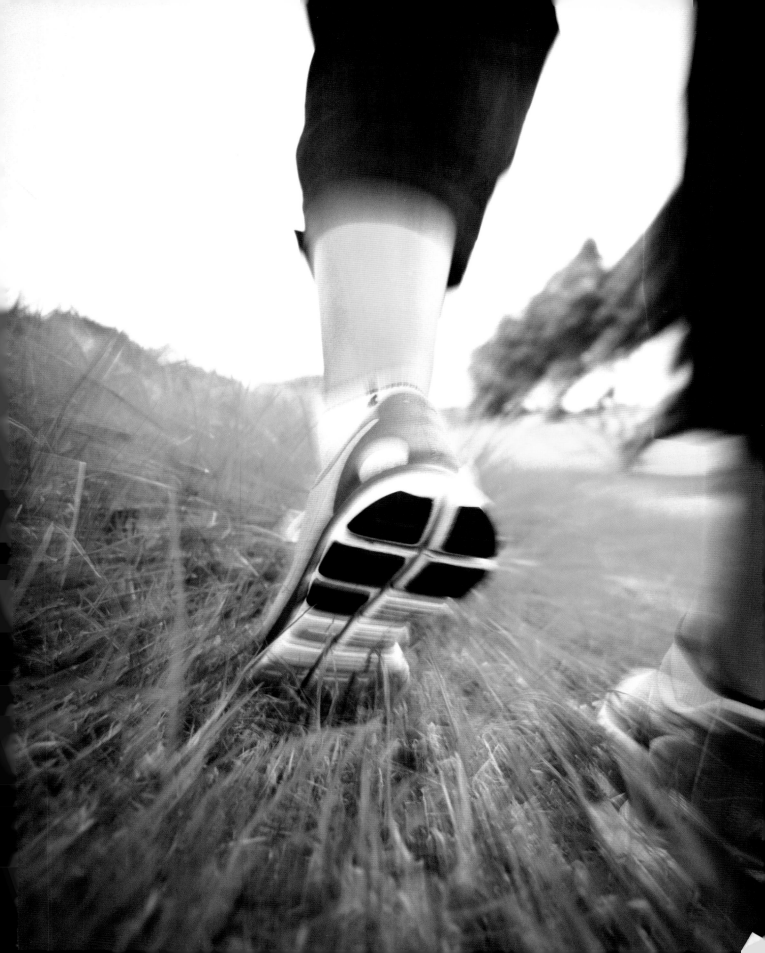

It's good to remember:
Pick an exercise you enjoy
and build it into your life in
a way that it becomes a habit
and a simple pleasure you
can't live without.

TARGET PRACTICE

Different forms of exercise have different targeted health benefits:

- Aerobic, such as skipping or circuit training—good for losing weight and getting fit.
- Flexibility, such as a yoga or stretch class—good for overall tone and flexibility, and helps to loosen your joints.
- Resistance, such as lifting weights at the gym—increases muscle mass and builds lean body mass, but even lifting the washing basket to the line and pegging it up, carrying the shopping and lifting the baby is a form of resistance exercise—especially as they get bigger. Don't accept help from a chivalrous husband or son; if it's a safe weight, do it yourself.

Sticking to your steps

Motivation is, for many, the most difficult part of maintaining a regular exercise routine. We are all motivated by different things, so it can help to find what it is that motivates you. The feeling of wellbeing that exercise promotes is a common motivator. For others, it's wanting to keep up with the kids or grandchildren, or be a good role model. Getting back to or keeping in shape is important. If you are a busy parent, exercise can be the one thing you can give yourself as 'time out'. We know that people who plan exercise daily are more likely to do it most days of the week, and that people who exercise in the morning are less likely to be waylaid by the day's pressing priorities. Some other things that help when it comes to motivation are:

- Exercise buddies.
- Joining a gym.
- Group exercise classes.
- Personal trainers.
- Daily tracking on a website.

If starting out is a problem for you, write a list of pros and cons, or make a list of the barriers you anticipate or the triggers that make you not want to exercise. Once you've done this, find solutions to overcome them. One great tip I learnt from my male patients is to set yourself up for success by registering in advance (alone or with a friend) for a boot camp, fun run or charity bike ride—a deadline that will keep you focused and is sure to get you started.

The good news is that your body gets used to exercise and it becomes a 'don't have to think about it' regular part of your day—to the point where your body will remind you and begin to insist that you 'just start'. You will begin to feel lost, lousy and incomplete without it.

When exercising is a problem

It is always important that when you exercise you don't overdo it. For example, walk at a pace where your breathing is increased but you can still talk and you're not out of breath. If you are trying too hard you may make it too arduous a task and it will become self-defeating—or worse, you may damage something.

For some, regular exercise appears impossible. If you are in poor health, you may need specialist advice to direct you towards small, gentle exercises, some even done while simply standing or sitting. Concentrate and build on what you can do and don't dwell on what you can't.

As always, if you have any health concerns or before you embark on a new exercise program, seek your doctor's advice.

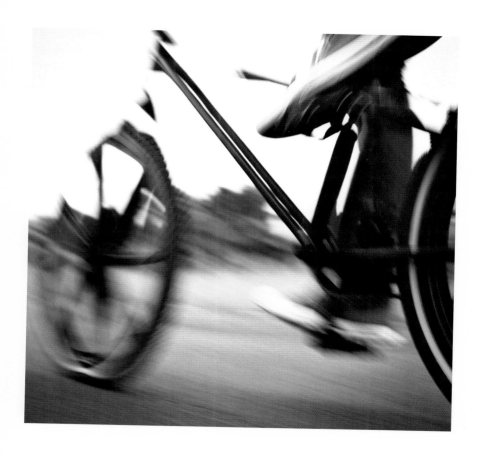

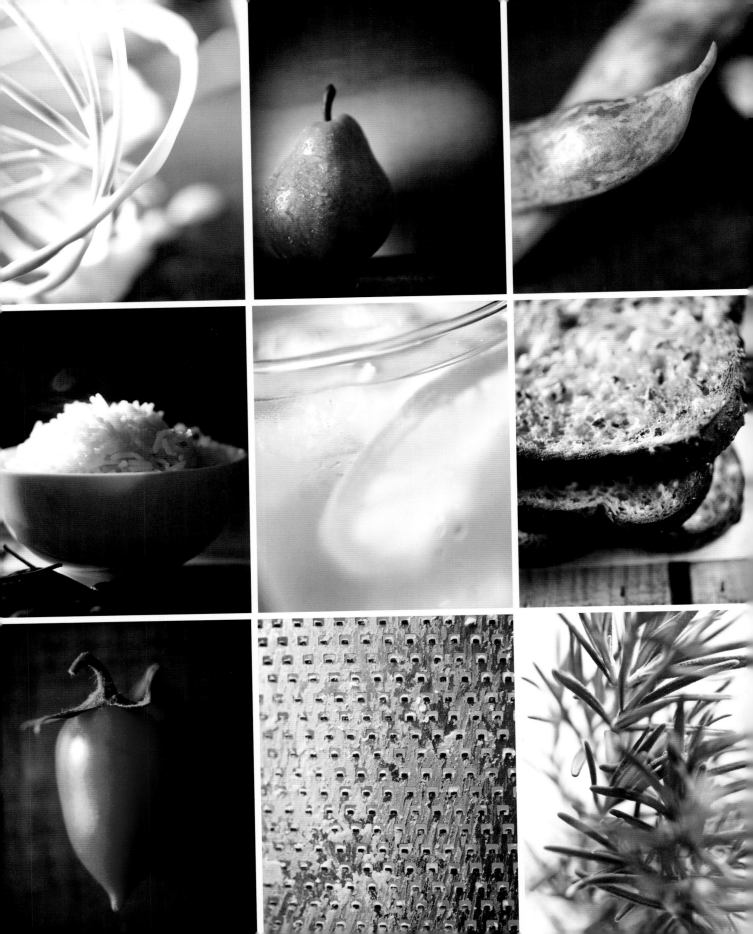

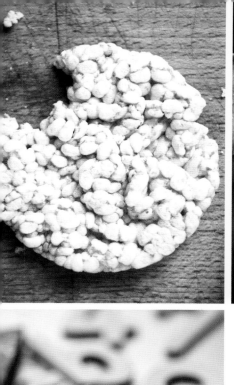
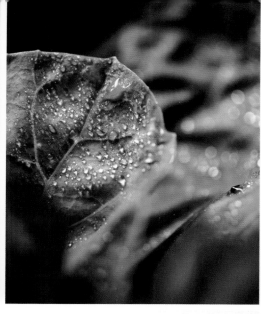
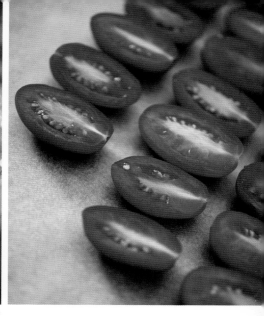
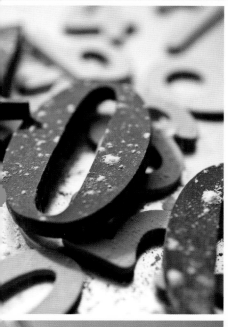
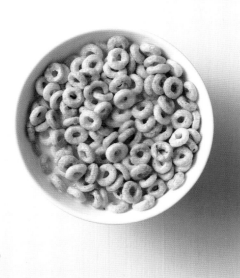

THE FOOD LOVER'S WAY TO A HAPPY WEIGHT

2

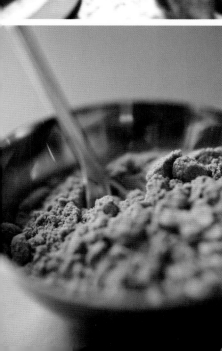
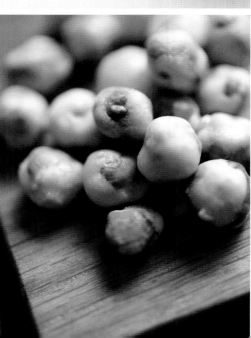
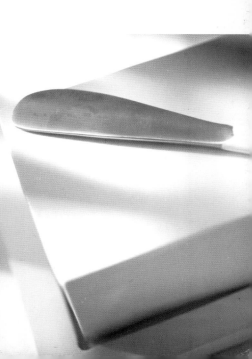

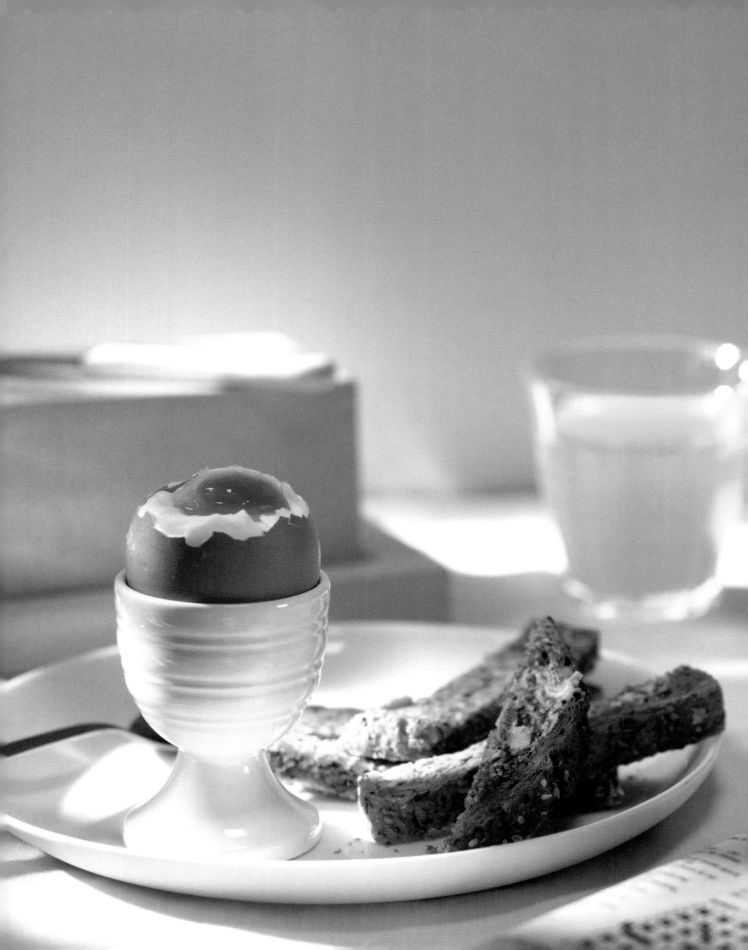

We want you to get the breakfast habit. It doesn't have to be a 'big deal, sit-down meal', but it's important to break the fast when counting your way to a healthy life. Whether you like waking up to cereal and fruit or a hearty cooked meal of eggs, toast and tomatoes, a good breakfast sets you up for the day ahead.

The food lover's way to a healthy breakfast

A good breakfast:

Kick-starts your metabolism.

Provides a steady supply of energy to help you stay alert and focused through the morning.

Keeps hunger pangs at bay and reduces the tendency to snack.

Helps you maintain a healthy weight. It's true: regular breakfast eaters tend to be slimmer than those who skip it.

It's good to remember: Make sure the first thing you eat each day is breakfast. It's the most important meal of the day. A satisfying breakfast will have about 10 to 25 counts.

Q&A

Q: I am trying to diet. I find it really easy to skip breakfast to cut counts as I'm not really that hungry first thing and can easily wait until midmorning and have an organic blueberry muffin from the canteen. And that keeps me going until my lunch break, which is around 1 p.m. Will this help me lose weight?

A: Skipping breakfast does not help with weight loss. Regular breakfast eaters are more likely to maintain a healthy weight than those who don't regularly eat breakfast. Often people compensate for missing breakfast by eating more snacks—usually fatty and sugary ones—during the day. So, if you are losing weight, you'll be more likely to keep the kilos off if you eat breakfast every day. Fibre- and wholegrain-rich breakfasts can be a great way to fill you up while helping to keep the counts down.

Q: It's really a rush at my place in the mornings, with school lunches to make, uniforms to iron and four of us to get out of the door by 8 a.m. No wonder I'm tired by the time I get to my desk at 9 a.m. How do I find time to eat breakfast?

A: We all have those mornings when there just isn't time to grab something to eat before we leave home. The key thing to remember is you should always try to eat something in the morning for breakfast (when you get to work, if that suits you better), so you are not craving a high-count snack by 11 a.m. Think about it—you wouldn't go to work or hit the school run without brushing your teeth or washing your face, so why start the morning without nourishing your body? Here are a few rush-hour breakfast tips:

- Prepare some bircher muesli or chopped fruit the night before, pre-pack it in an airtight container and store it in the fridge so you can grab it on your way to work.
- Keep a bowl, spoon and cereal at work—cereal and milk is one of the quickest breakfasts there is.
- Pick up a 'cereal in a cup' from your local supermarket—all you need to do is add milk!
- Grab a slice of wholemeal toast with Vegemite and combine it with a tub of fruity low-fat or diet yoghurt for those off-site early morning meetings.
- Crunch into an apple or have a single-serve tub of fruit and some yoghurt.
- Just remember, if time is limited and breakfast is rushed, top up the wholegrain or whatever you've missed, at other meals.

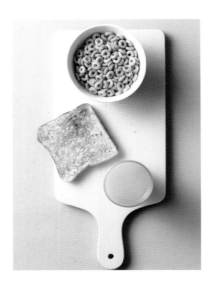

It's good to remember:
Don't miss out on the good things in life. Have breakfast.

I'm not hungry

If you're not hungry when you first wake up, keep something at work to eat when you arrive. Going without breakfast sets you on a downward spiral for the rest of the day.

I need my sleep—that extra half-hour makes a difference

A banana takes just a minute or two to peel and eat. Cereal and milk is quick and easy. Choose wholegrain, ready-to-eat, crispy breakfast cereals (such as CHEERIOS or VITA BRITS), or natural muesli. They are typically low in fat and are an important source of vitamins and minerals, a good source of fibre and a lower sugar choice. Just add skim or reduced-fat milk for a healthy breakfast.

I have a really early start

If you're up really early, plan ways to include breakfast foods a little later in the morning (at morning tea, even)—just don't starve yourself of those important nutrients and energy.

I hate breakfast foods

You don't have to eat breakfast foods at breakfast. But you do need to 'break the fast' because, while you were tucked up in bed enjoying a good night's sleep, your body was still hard at work breathing, regulating your body temperature and repairing your body cells. All this seemingly effortless activity burns fuel, so your body's fuel tank will be hovering around empty come morning.

Excuse buster

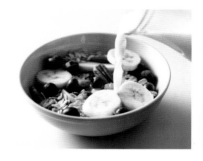

Get a boost from a banana and get the energy working for you. Peel and eat or mash, dice or slice, and serve with cereal and fruit.

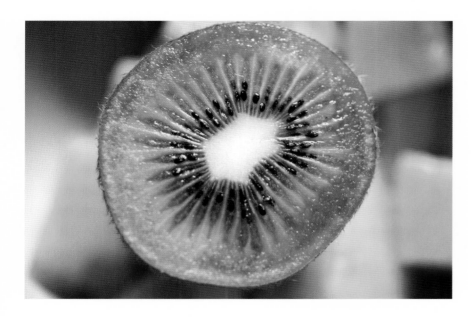

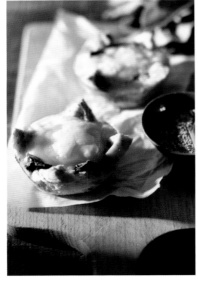

It's good to remember:
Here's how the counts add up when you get the frying pan out: two eggs (10) + two thin slices of toast (6) + two rashers of bacon (11) + ¾ cup orange juice (4) = 31 counts. If adding a spray of oil, add 2 counts.

Healthy breakfasts you can count on

Nourish your body, boost your fibre intake and power your day with the right fuel at breakfast time. Aim for 10–20 counts for breakfast, depending on how hungry you are first thing in the morning. Check out the counts for some typical breakfasts below:

13 counts

- An omelet made with two large eggs, ⅓ cup of full-cream milk, chopped shallots (spring onions) to taste and 2 tablespoons of diced tomato. OR
- Sliced mushrooms (70g) gently sautéed in 1 tablespoon of olive oil and topped with lots of fresh parsley, served on toasted Turkish bread (5x11cm).

14 counts

- A bowl of porridge (made with ½ cup of raw oats) with ½ cup of full-cream milk and topped with 2 tablespoons of sultanas, plus a cup of tea with milk.

15 counts

- Two pieces of thin wholegrain toast, each spread with 1 teaspoon of margarine and a smear of Vegemite, plus ¾ cup of reduced-fat milk.
- An English muffin split in half, toasted and topped with ⅓ cup of reduced-fat ricotta cheese, tomato slices and a few twists of freshly ground black pepper.
- A medium pancake topped with ⅓ cup of reduced-fat ricotta and a drizzle of honey, served with a glass of water.

16 counts

- Two VITA BRITS, ½ cup of reduced-fat milk, one small banana and ¾ cup of orange juice. OR
- A 200ml tub of reduced-fat yoghurt topped with ½ cup of granola with a single-serve tub of diced fruit and a drizzle of honey.

17 counts

- ⅓ cup of Swiss muesli with ½ cup of reduced-fat milk, one small sliced banana and a cup of green tea.

18 counts

- A round of wholemeal sourdough toast scraped with margarine, topped with a poached egg, two slices of smoked salmon cut into strips and a little chopped dill, plus a glass of water.

Build a better breakfast (with cereal and toast)

Most of us opt for cereal or toast for brekkie most days. However, as easy as that sounds, the bread and cereal aisles in the supermarket are packed with options all claiming to be 'healthy'. So which to choose? Here's how you can take charge and build a better breakfast in 5 minutes.

Priority # 1: Portion size counts

When making breakfast (or ordering it in a café or canteen), portion size counts—the bigger the portion, the more counts you'll be totting up. But it's also important to have a satisfying brekkie so that you're not craving a high-count midmorning snack. Here are some typical portions that will satisfy most people at breakfast time. (Counts are shown on page 48.)

- ⅓ cup (about 45g) of natural (untoasted) muesli.
- Two wheat- or oat-flake biscuits like VITA BRITS.
- 1 cup (about 30g) of crispy, ready-to-eat wholegrain cereal like CHEERIOS.
- ½ cup of raw porridge oats (makes 1 cup cooked porridge).
- Two thin (sandwich bread) slices or one slice of thick (not double-thick) wholegrain bread.

Priority # 2: Make it wholegrain

In the supermarket, make the switch to 'wholegrain' breakfast cereals and breads. Unlike refined grains, wholegrains deliver a nutritious package of the complete grain—the bran, endosperm and germ. Including more wholegrains in your meals and snacks is a key ingredient in the recipe for health and wellbeing.

Priority # 3: Focus on fibre

Check the nutrition label and make sure the cereal you start your day with has at least 3g of fibre per serving, and that the bread you pop into the toaster has at least 1.5g of fibre per slice. More is better. Fibre-rich breakfasts fill you up while keeping the counts down and, of course, help you on your way to your 30g of fibre a day.

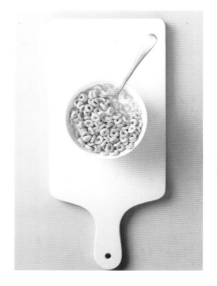

It's good to remember: Get into a daily habit with fibre-rich wholegrains.

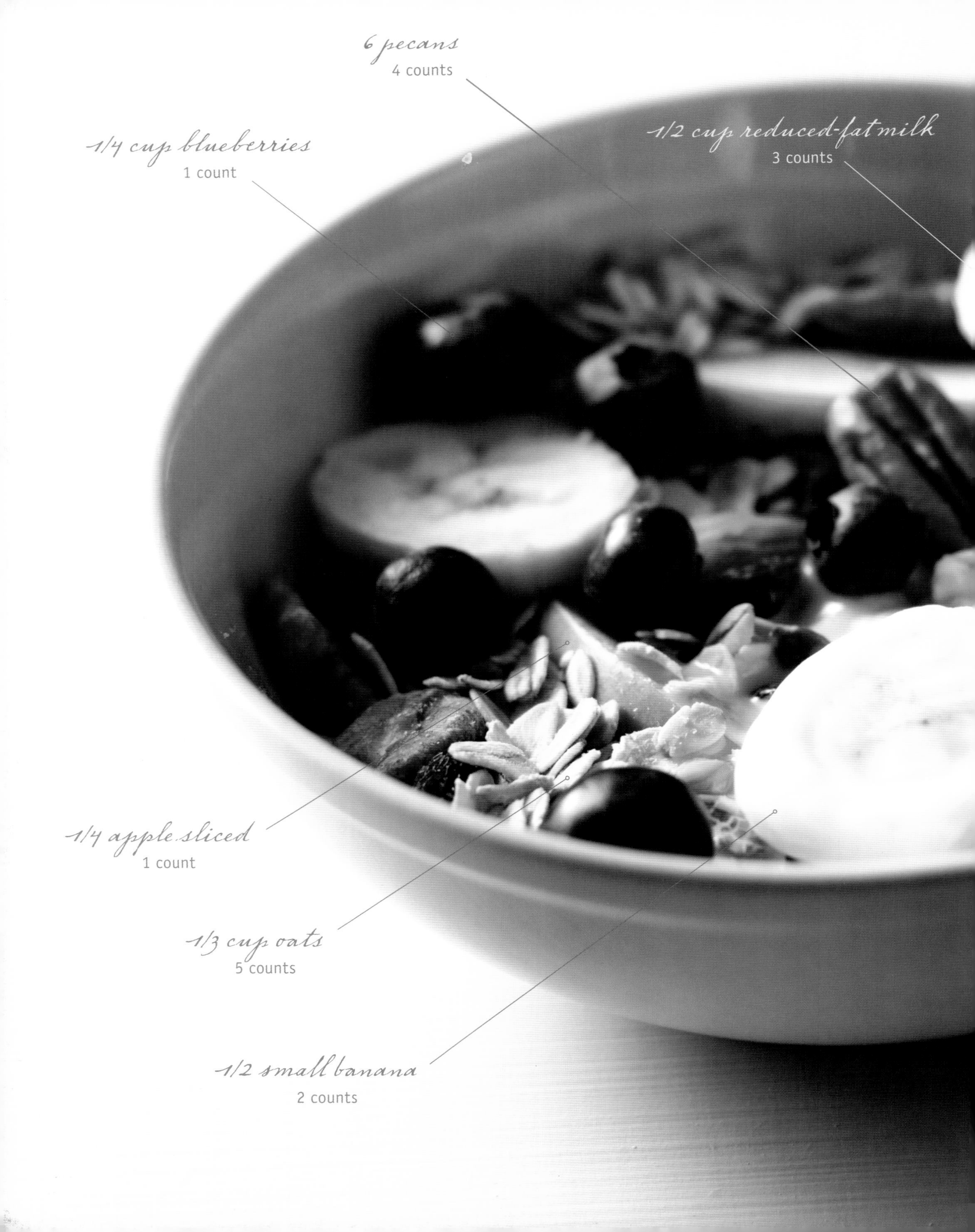

6 pecans
4 counts

1/4 cup blueberries
1 count

1/2 cup reduced-fat milk
3 counts

1/4 apple sliced
1 count

1/3 cup oats
5 counts

1/2 small banana
2 counts

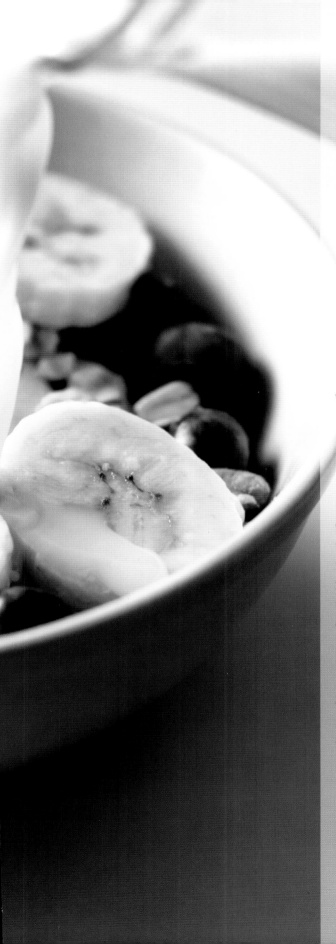

Know your oats

What's so 'super' about a bowl of oats?

- Good source of fibre.
- 100% wholegrain.
- Provides vitamins, minerals and antioxidants.
- No added sugar or salt.

Oats contain both insoluble and soluble fibres. But they are especially rich in a particular type of soluble fibre called beta-glucan. This fibre absorbs fluids, forming a gel-like solution in our tummies, helping us feel fuller for longer but also helping to lower cholesterol reabsorption.

Seriously oaty cereals include UNCLE TOBYS Oats, OATBRITS, OAT CRISP, MORNING SUN Muesli, oat muesli bars and even a tablespoon or two of natural oat bran. Combine them with an oat-based snack later in the day if you or anyone in your family could benefit from eating more oats.

It's good to remember:
Build healthy bones with
some servings of dairy
food every day.

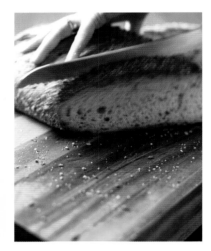

Mix and match your breakfast

Here are our top tips for putting together a healthy breakfast:

- ✔ Have some form of dairy food or a dairy alternative for calcium, vitamins, minerals and protein—and one of your daily serves.
- ✔ Switch to a wholegrain and high-fibre cereal or grainy bread as your main source of carbohydrates. Quality carbohydrates should provide fibre and a long-lasting source of energy, so you continue to feel satisfied several hours after eating.
- ✔ Add in some fruit—be it fresh, canned, frozen or dried—for one of your daily serves.
- ✔ Feel fuller for longer by including protein foods with your breakfast—a handful of nuts or seeds on your cereal, a serving of dairy food, or an egg or baked beans.
- ✔ Don't forget a drink to stay hydrated.

To kick-start the day, a good breakfast will have around 10–20 counts. The counts we give here are only average counts for these typical foods. Check out the counts for your favourite foods in our ready-reckoner (page 222).

Typical counts for breads and grains

- **3 counts** = one thin slice of wholegrain bread; one small pancake (8cm); one wheat- or oat-flake breakfast biscuit.
- **4 counts** = one wholemeal crumpet; one small bagel; one slice of fruit loaf or raisin bread; ½ cup of creamed corn; half an English muffin.
- **5 counts** = ½ cup of cooked rice (brown or white); one thick (toast) slice of wholegrain bread; one thick slice of soy and linseed bread; one medium pancake (10cm).
- **6 counts** = one slice of heavy fruit bread; one breakfast cereal bar; 1 cup of ready-to-eat, crispy wholegrain breakfast cereal; one flavoured sachet of instant oats.
- **7 counts** = one English-style multigrain muffin; one medium bagel; 1 cup of cooked porridge.
- **8 counts** = one double-thick slice of wholegrain bread; ⅓ cup of natural muesli.
- **9 counts** = one spicy fruit English muffin; ⅓ cup of toasted muesli.
- **11 counts** = one large bagel.
- **12 counts** = one large pancake (12cm); one large waffle.

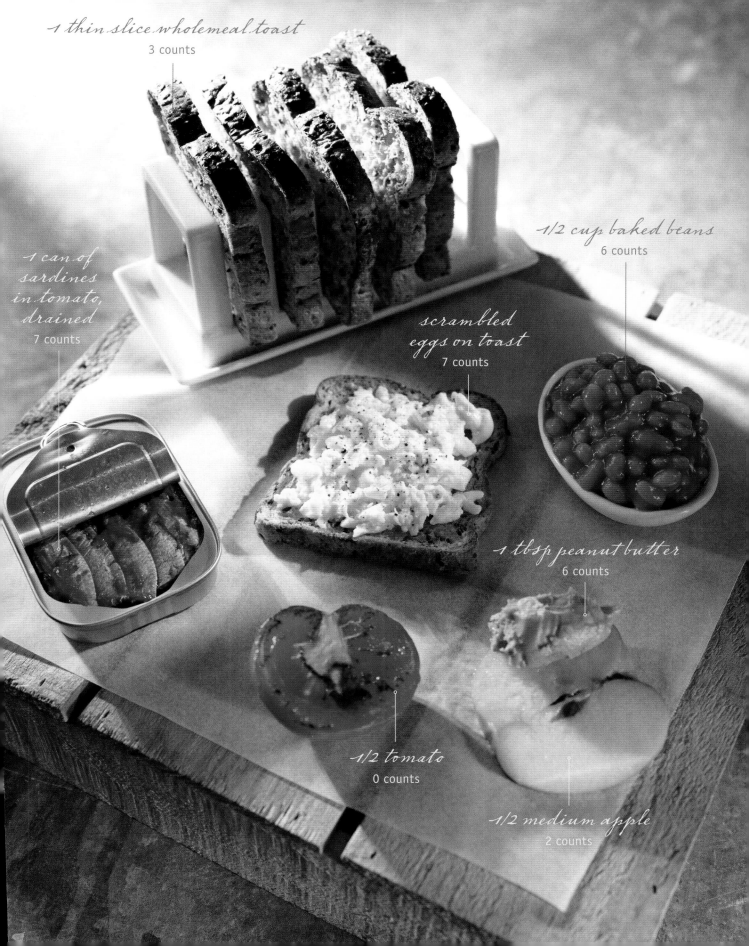

1 thin slice wholemeal toast
3 counts

1/2 cup baked beans
6 counts

1 can of sardines in tomato, drained
7 counts

scrambled eggs on toast
7 counts

1 tbsp peanut butter
6 counts

1/2 tomato
0 counts

1/2 medium apple
2 counts

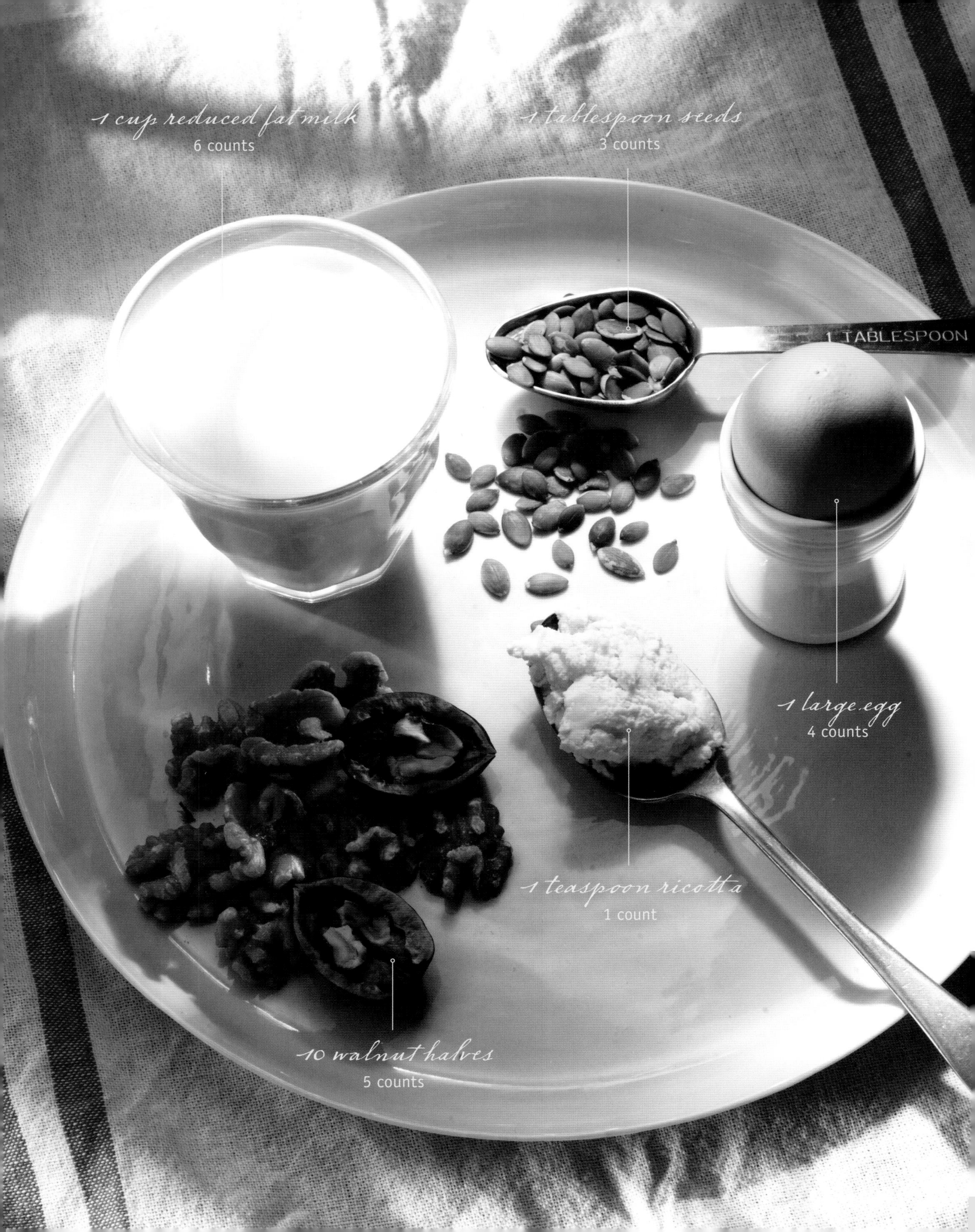

1 cup reduced fat milk
6 counts

1 tablespoon seeds
3 counts

1 large egg
4 counts

1 teaspoon ricotta
1 count

10 walnut halves
5 counts

1 TABLESPOON

Typical counts for eggs, dairy foods, nuts and seeds, legumes, meat and fish

- **1 count** = 1 tablespoon of cottage cheese or ricotta; one slice of smoked salmon.
- **2 counts** = ½ cup of reduced-fat or skim milk; half a tub (200g) of diet yoghurt; 100g soft/silken tofu; two slices (30g) of smoked salmon.
- **3 counts** = one medium (47g) egg (boiled or poached); ten almonds; 1 tablespoon of sunflower seeds; 1 tablespoon of LSA.
- **4 counts** = ½ cup of full-cream milk; half a tub (200g) of low-fat flavoured yoghurt (added sugar); one large (53g) egg (boiled or poached or scrambled with 1 tablespoon of skim milk); 1 tablespoon of pepitas.
- **5 counts** = half a tub (200g) of full-cream yoghurt; ½ cup of canned kidney or other beans, drained; 100g firm/hard tofu; one jumbo (67g) egg (boiled or poached); ten walnut halves; one rasher of cooked bacon; half a can (45g) of sardines in water or tomato sauce.
- **6 counts** = ½ cup of baked beans in tomato sauce; one thin grilled sausage.
- **7 counts** = ½ cup of baked beans in ham sauce.
- **10 counts** = one thick grilled sausage.

Typical counts for vegetables

- **0 counts** = baby spinach; sliced raw mushrooms; capsicum slices; grilled tomato halves; canned asparagus spears; tomato salsa; jarred artichokes or mushrooms (in brine).
- **2 counts** = ½ cup of canned mushrooms (in butter).
- **5 counts** = ½ cup of sautéed onion rings (in minimum oil).

Typical counts for fats and oils

- **1 count** = 1 tablespoon of mashed or one slice of avocado; 1 tablespoon of extra-light cream cheese.
- **2 counts** = 1 teaspoon of margarine or butter; 1 tablespoon of light cream cheese.
- **3 counts** = 1 tablespoon of full-fat cream cheese.
- **4 counts** = 2 teaspoons of olive oil; 1 tablespoon of cream.
- **5 counts** = half a small avocado.
- **6 counts** = 1 tablespoon of peanut butter (smooth, crunchy or light).

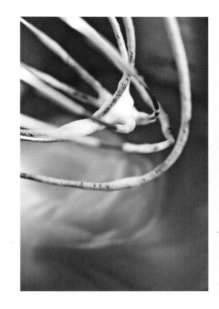

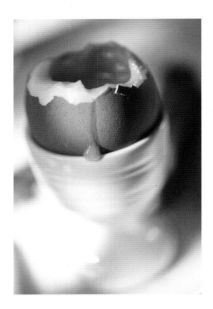

Eggs are a smart protein choice if weight control is important.

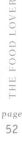
It's good to remember: When in doubt about what to order, use your phone app to help you count your options.

Typical counts for fruit

- **2 counts** = one medium mandarin; half a medium pawpaw (papaya), two large apricots; ½ cup of blueberries; 1 tablespoon of sultanas; five medium strawberries.
- **3 counts** = one medium kiwifruit; five large strawberries; one large peach or nectarine; two medium plums; 1 cup of pineapple cubes; one (3cm) thick slice of watermelon; ½ cup of stewed fruit (no sugar added); five medium dried apricots; three medium pitted dates; two dried figs.
- **4 counts** = 1 cup of fresh fruit salad; one medium apple; one small banana; one medium orange; one medium pear; ½ rockmelon; small bunch (22) grapes; ½ cup of canned fruit (in juice or water); four stewed prunes (without sugar).
- **5 counts** = 1 cup of fruit juice; ½ cup of stewed fruit (with added sugar); four stewed prunes (with sugar).

Keeping count when you're out

Everyone likes to eat breakfast out once in a while, so here are some key tips to help you make the right choices when running your eyes over the menu.

Start with lean protein. Good choices include skim milk (on cereal or in a latte or cappuccino), low-fat yoghurt, low-fat cheese, or eggs (hard-boiled, poached or scrambled in non-fat spray).

Go wholegrain for your breads and cereals. We all need a variety of fibre-rich foods in our daily diet. That means wholegrain breads and cereals, or wholemeal or buckwheat pancakes.

Order fruitful dishes. Fruit is a goldmine of vitamins, minerals, fibre and health-giving antioxidants. Grapefruit halves, melon slices and seasonal fruit salads are tasty options.

Load up on calcium. Fat-free or low-fat milk, or milk-based foods are a terrific source of calcium, vital for building and maintaining healthy bones and teeth. Enjoy coffee drinks like latte that are made with lots of milk, or yoghurt or a bowl of cereal with milk. Smoothies can be a calcium-rich option—but keep an eye on portion size and extra counts.

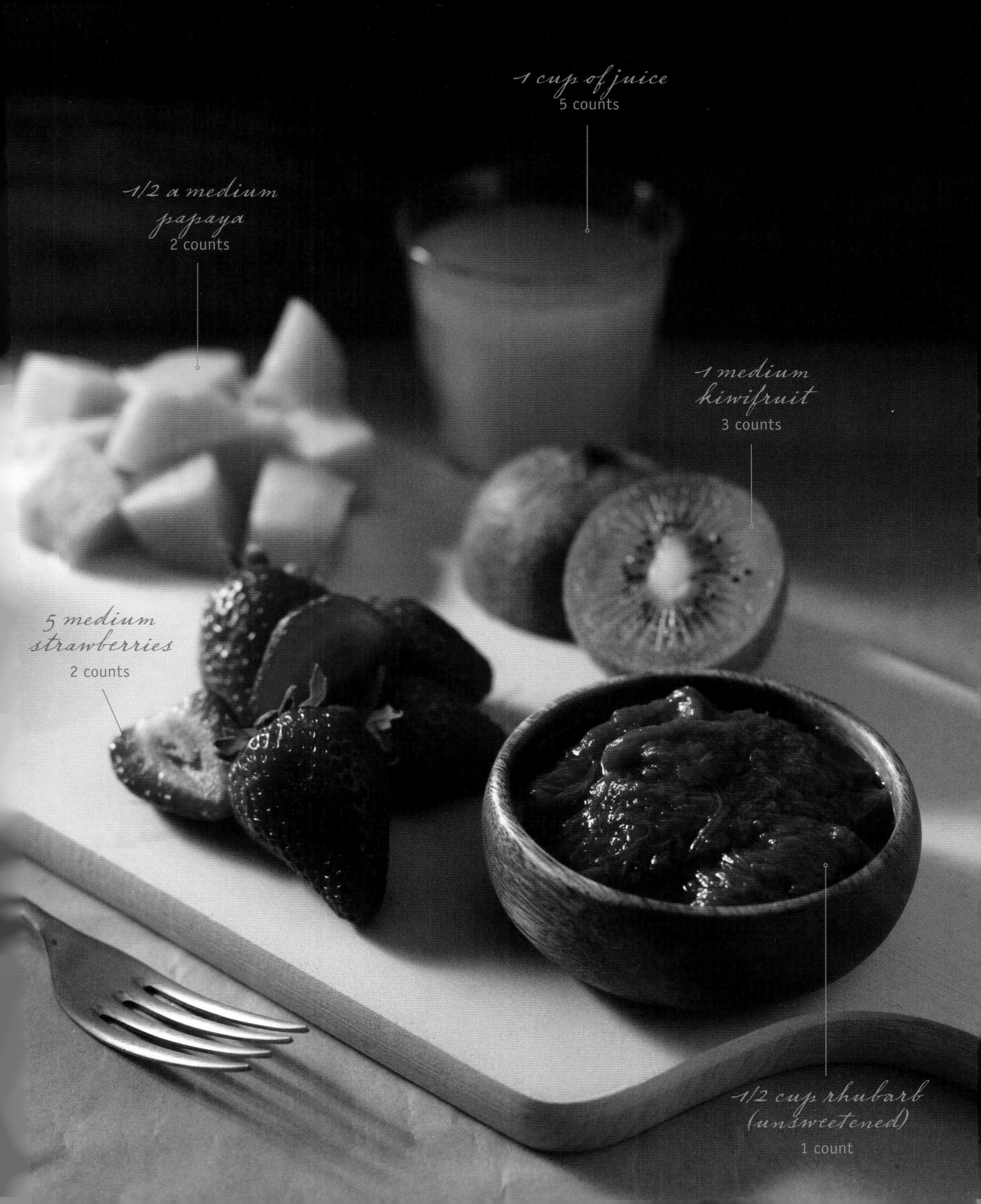

1 cup of juice
5 counts

1/2 a medium
papaya
2 counts

1 medium
kiwifruit
3 counts

5 medium
strawberries
2 counts

1/2 cup rhubarb
(unsweetened)
1 count

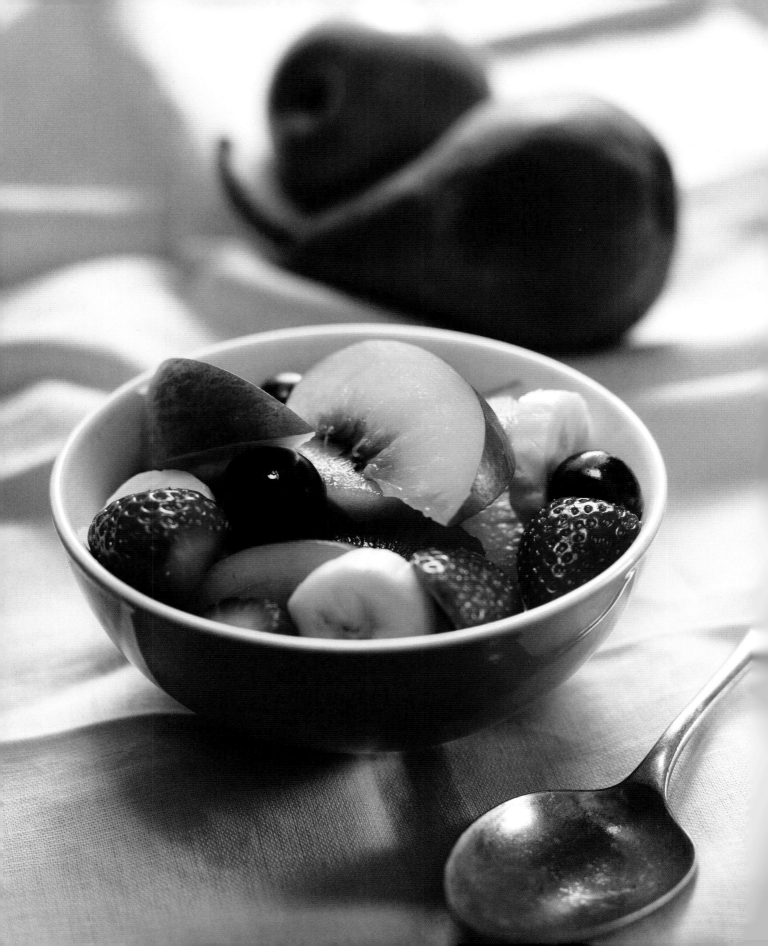

Healthy breakfast recipes

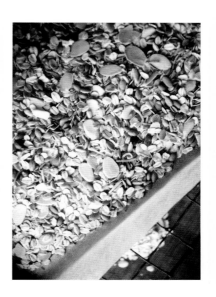

DIY muesli

½ cup UNCLE TOBYS Traditional Oats

½ cup wholegrain barley flakes

2 shredded wheat biscuits, crushed

2 tbsp coarsely chopped brazil nuts

2 tbsp coarsely chopped hazelnuts

2 tbsp sunflower seeds

⅓ cup coarsely chopped dried apricots

1 Mix together the muesli ingredients in a large bowl, then spoon into a clean, airtight container and store in a cool, dry place.

This muesli recipe will keep for up to two weeks in an airtight container, so make double the quantity, or even more if you wish. You can vary the nuts, seeds and dried fruit—the counts will be similar as long as you keep the quantities the same. Serve with seasonal fresh fruit, or with canned fruit and low-fat milk or yoghurt if you wish.

PREP: 10 mins

SERVES: 4

COUNTS PER SERVE: 12

¼ CUP LOW-FAT MILK: 2 counts

PREP: 10 mins
SERVES: 4
COUNTS PER SERVE: 19

Bircher muesli

2 cups UNCLE TOBYS Traditional Oats

½ cup low-fat milk

1 cup apple juice

1 tbsp lemon juice

2 tbsp honey

½ cup dried apricots, chopped

4 fresh dates, pitted and quartered

1 green apple, grated

½ cup low-fat natural yoghurt

1 In a large bowl combine the oats, milk, juices, honey, apricots and dates. Cover and leave in the fridge overnight.
2 In the morning, fold through the apple and yoghurt, and serve.

We made this with apple, but it's just as delicious with pears. Make it with your favourite flavoured yoghurt, but choose low fat to keep the counts down.

PREP: 5 mins
SERVES: 2
COUNTS PER SERVE: 12

Fruity cereal delight

2 cups CHEERIOS

200g tub low-fat vanilla yoghurt

1 medium apple, sliced into slivers

2 tbsp sultanas or raisins

1 Arrange the ingredients in two glasses or dishes in alternating layers of CHEERIOS, yoghurt, apple slices and sultanas.

Oat and macadamia granola topping

1 cup UNCLE TOBYS Traditional Oats

⅓ cup sunflower seeds

⅓ cup slivered almonds

½ cup coarsely chopped macadamia nuts

2 tbsp honey

1 tbsp raw sugar

1 Preheat the oven to 150°C.

2 Combine the oats, seeds and nuts in a baking dish, and bake for 20 minutes or until golden.

3 Remove from the oven, stir through the honey and sugar, making sure they are well-combined, then bake for a further 10 minutes.

4 Set aside to cool, then spoon into a clean, airtight container and store in a cool, dry place.

You need to use traditional rolled oats to give you the right texture for this nutty topping. Sprinkle 1 tablespoon over fresh, poached or canned fruit or yoghurt, or on a creamy bowl of porridge. It also makes a delicious crunchy topping for desserts.

PREP: 5 mins

COOK: 30 mins

SERVES: about 30 x 1 tbsp

COUNTS PER SERVE: 1

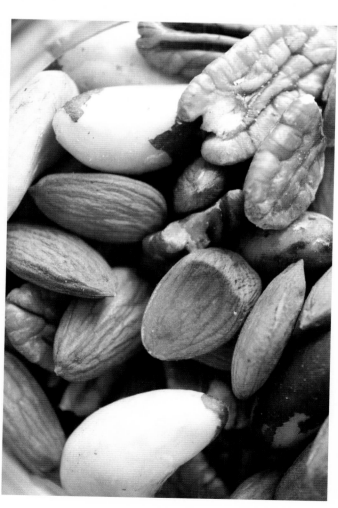

PREP: 10 mins
COOK: 10 mins
SERVES: 4
COUNTS PER SERVE: 11

Spicy citrus and berry fruits

¾ cup water

½ cup caster sugar

1 cinnamon stick

6 whole cloves

1 lemon, juiced and zested

1 lime, juiced and zested

4 oranges, segmented

1 cup mixed berries

2 x 200g tubs diet vanilla yoghurt

1 Combine the water, sugar, cinnamon, cloves, lemon and lime in a large pan and bring to the boil. Turn the heat down and simmer for 10 minutes to reduce the syrup to ¾ cup, then strain the liquid and leave it to cool.

2 Divide fruits into four bowls, and top with the prepared syrup and yoghurt.

A smoothie can be a real energy booster in the morning. Experiment with different fruits in season or use canned fruits (in juice or water and drained) if you prefer. Try different flavours of low-fat or diet yoghurts to change the flavour, too. For those who are lactose intolerant, the milk and yoghurt can be replaced with soy milk and yoghurt, but try to use calcium-enriched and low-fat varieties.

PREP: 5 mins
SERVES: 2
COUNTS PER SERVE: 10

Creamy banana smoothie

1 cup skim milk

200g tub low-fat vanilla yoghurt

2 tbsp skim milk powder

2 tbsp wheatgerm or oat bran

1 large ripe banana, peeled

1 Combine all the ingredients in a blender, process until frothy and smooth, and serve immediately.

Variations

• Strawberry smoothie—replace the banana with ½ cup of hulled strawberries (9 counts).

• Peach smoothie—replace the banana with one large peeled and stoned peach (10 counts).

• Mango smoothie—replace the banana with one small mango, peeled and sliced (11 counts).

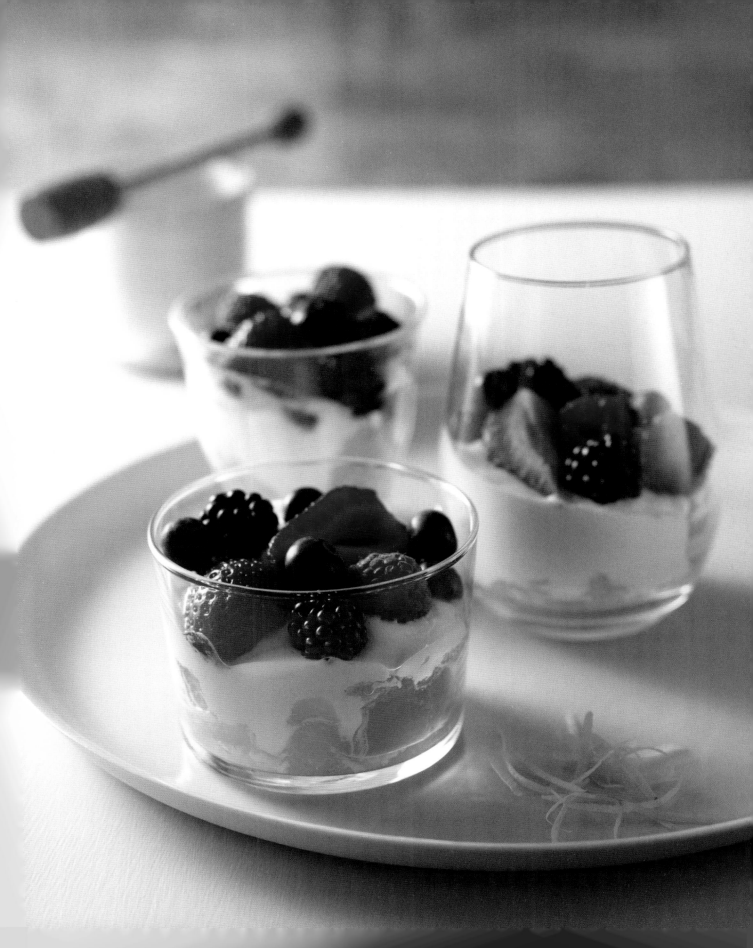

Add any nuts you like to this recipe. LSA (a ground product that contains linseeds, sunflower seeds and almonds) is also great to include when making porridge.

PREP: 5 mins
COOK: 10 mins
SERVES: 4
COUNTS PER SERVE: 15

Nutty porridge

Nutty topping

½ cup UNCLE TOBYS Traditional Oats
½ cup roughly chopped mixed nuts such as macadamias, pistachios
  and almonds
2 tsp honey

Porridge

1 cup UNCLE TOBYS Traditional Oats
½ cup chopped dried fruit
2½ cups cold water

1 Preheat the grill (medium heat).
2 To make the topping, mix the oats, nuts and honey together, and spread over a baking tray. Place under the grill and cook until crisp and lightly golden, stirring occasionally.
3 To make the porridge, combine the oats, dried fruit and water in a saucepan, and stir well. Place over high heat and bring to the boil. Reduce the heat and simmer gently for 5 minutes until the oats are thick and creamy.
4 Divide between serving bowls, sprinkle the topping over each and serve immediately.

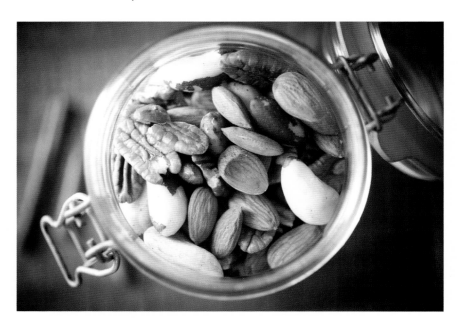

Cornjacks with fresh tomato salsa

Fresh tomato salsa

2 large ripe tomatoes, diced

¼ cup chopped fresh coriander leaves

1 tbsp extra virgin olive oil

zest and juice of 1 lime

Cornjacks

¾ cup cornmeal polenta

¼ tsp bicarbonate of soda

¼ cup plain flour

1½ tbsp margarine, melted

¼ cup CARNATION Light & Creamy Evaporated Milk

½ cup corn kernels

4 shallots (spring onions), chopped

canola oil spray

1 Prepare the salsa by combining all the salsa ingredients in a bowl.

2 For the cornjacks, combine the polenta, bicarbonate of soda and flour in a bowl, and make a well in the centre. Pour in the melted margarine, evaporated milk, corn kernels and shallots, and stir until combined.

3 Spray a non-stick pan with oil spray and cook tablespoonfuls of corn mixture until the top has set. Turn and brown the other side.

4 Serve hot with a dollop of salsa.

Serve these with tomatoes—the tomato salsa below, fresh tomato slices drizzled with a little balsamic vinegar, tiny cherry tomatoes cut into halves and sprinkled with a little freshly ground black pepper, or grilled tomato halves. These cornjacks are also great on their own with a dash of sweet chilli sauce. In the unlikely event there are leftovers, pop them into the lunch box.

PREP: 5 mins

COOK: 10 mins

SERVES: 4

COUNTS PER SERVE CORNJACKS: 13

COUNTS PER SERVE SALSA: 3

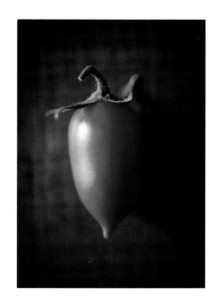

French toast with berry compote

Enjoy this berry compote
on French toast using your
favourite fresh or frozen
berries—strawberries,
raspberries, blackberries
or blueberries.

PREP: 5 mins
COOK: 15 mins
SERVES: 4
COUNTS PER SERVE: 10
TWO SERVES (ILLUSTRATED): 20

1 cup mixed berries

2 eggs

2 tbsp low-fat milk

4 slices fruit and muesli bread or fruit loaf, preferably wholegrain

2 tbsp pure maple syrup

1 Put the berries in a small saucepan and gently heat until the berries
   are warm and have softened.
2 Meanwhile, break the eggs into a flat dish, add milk and whisk with
   a fork to combine. Add slices of bread and coat well with the egg
   mixture on both sides.
3 Heat a non-stick frying pan over medium heat and dry-fry two slices
   of bread at a time for about 3 minutes on each side, or until golden.
   Repeat with remaining two slices.
4 Cut bread in half and serve topped with the warm berries and
   2 teaspoons of maple syrup drizzled over the top.

Creamy mushrooms on grainy toast

This creamy café favourite
is easy to make at home.
Serve with grilled tomatoes
and rocket, and really
make inroads on your
daily vegetable serves. You
need to use a very grainy
bread for this—it boosts
the flavour and the fibre.

PREP: 5 mins
COOK: 12 mins
SERVES: 4
COUNTS PER SERVE: 10

2 tsp olive oil

400g Swiss brown mushrooms, quartered

½ cup CARNATION Light & Creamy Evaporated Milk

1 packet mushroom soup mix

4 slices grainy 'toast' thickness bread

¼ cup flat-leaf parsley, leaves roughly chopped

1 Heat the oil in a deep-sided non-stick frying pan and cook the
   mushrooms for about 2 minutes.
2 In a small bowl, combine the evaporated milk and soup mix, then
   add to the mushrooms in the pan. Bring just to the boil, then reduce
   the heat and simmer gently for 7–10 minutes until thick, stirring
   constantly. Meanwhile, toast the bread.
3 Serve the mushrooms on toast topped with the fresh parsley.

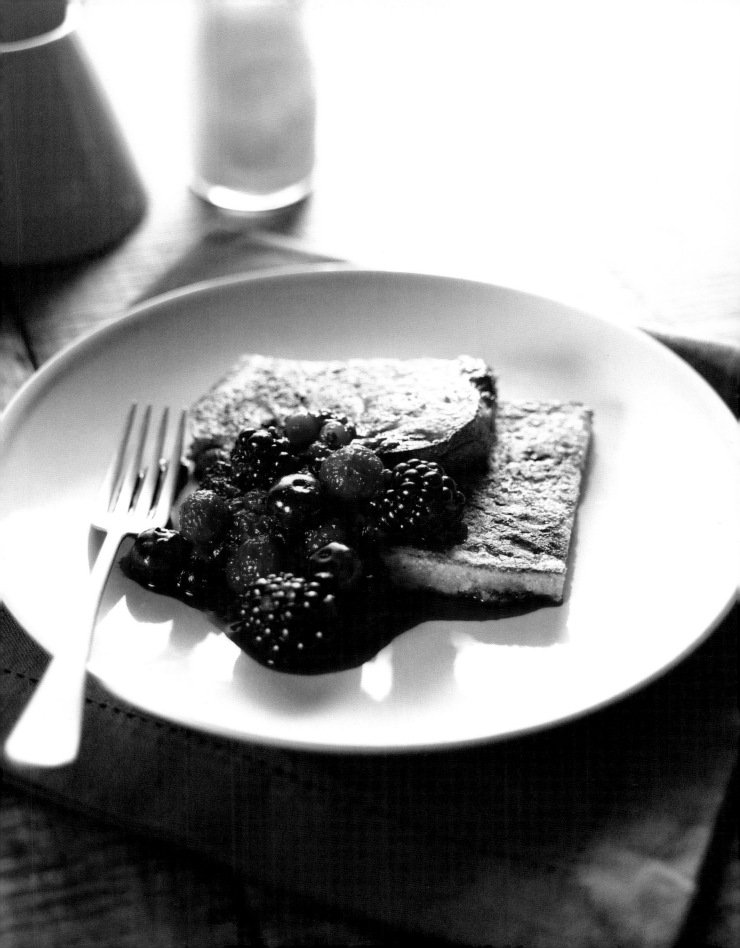

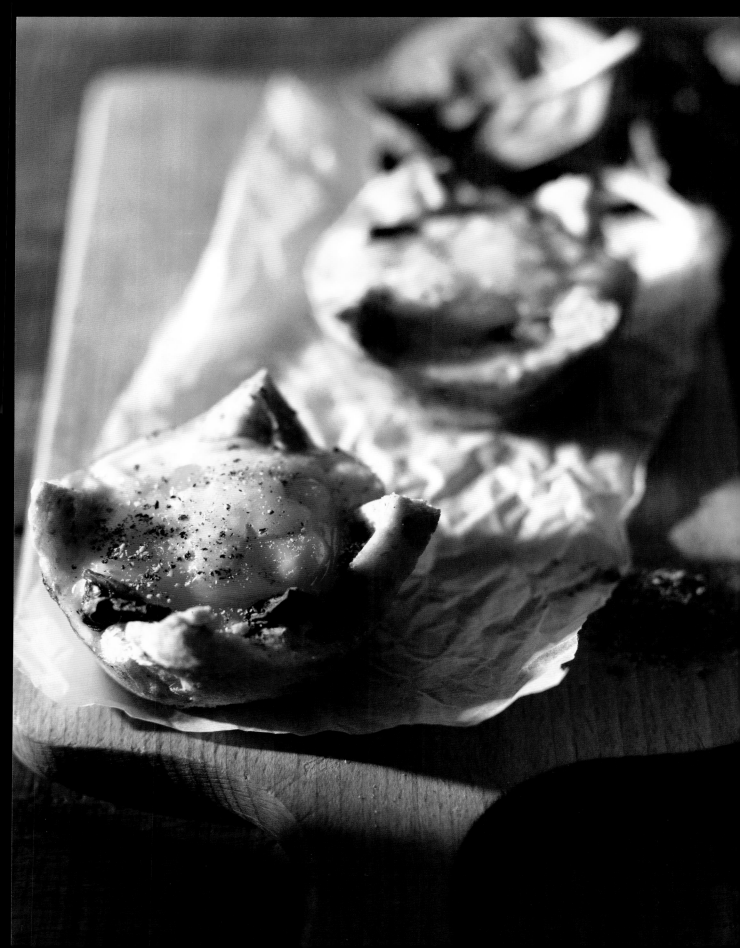

Eggs in nests

2 slices wholemeal or multigrain 'sandwich' bread

olive oil cooking spray

1 tsp olive oil margarine

4 button mushrooms, sliced and stems trimmed

3 English (not baby) spinach leaves, washed and chopped

freshly ground black pepper, to taste

2 eggs

1 tbsp coarsely grated, reduced-fat cheddar cheese

1 Preheat the oven to 180°C (160°C fan-forced).

2 Cut the crusts off the bread. Spray both sides of each slice lightly with oil. Press the bread slices firmly into two ⅓-cup capacity non-stick muffin pan holes. Set aside.

3 Heat the margarine in a non-stick frying pan over medium-high heat until sizzling. Add the mushrooms and cook, stirring often, for 4–5 minutes, or until tender. Add the spinach and cook, stirring, for 1–2 minutes, or until wilted. Remove from the heat and season with pepper.

4 Divide the mushroom mixture between the bread cases. Crack an egg into a small dish and then slide it into one of the bread cases. Repeat with the remaining egg. Sprinkle with the cheese. For a softly set yolk, bake for 15 minutes; for a hard-cooked yolk, 20 minutes.

5 Serve warm or at room temperature.

There are no breakfast skippers when nest eggs are on the menu. Children of all ages love them. And if you cook them until the yolk is firm, they are portable for people who need to rush out the door. Or you can save them for a lazy weekend breakfast or brunch when the family is a little more relaxed. Just make double the quantity for four people. This recipe could be gluten free if made with gluten-free bread.

PREP: 15 mins
COOK: 15–20 mins
SERVES: 2 (one 'nest' each)
COUNTS PER SERVE: 11

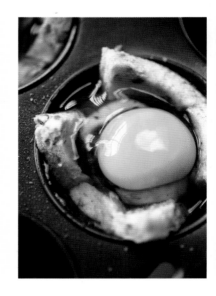

Pie apricot and pie apple can be found on the supermarket shelves with the other canned fruits. Making mini-sized muffins and cooking without fat (using pie fruit instead) keeps the counts down with these delicious muffins.

PREP: 10 mins
COOK: 20 mins
MAKES: 24
COUNTS PER SERVE: 7

Muesli breakfast mini muffins

1¼ cups UNCLE TOBYS Traditional Oats

2 cups self-raising flour

2 large eggs, lightly beaten

¼ cup brown sugar

1 cup milk

400g pie apricot or pie apple

1 Preheat the oven to 200°C (180°C fan-forced). Lightly grease two twelve-hole (⅓ cup) muffin tins.
2 Combine 1 cup of the oats with the flour, eggs, sugar, milk and pie apple in a bowl and mix well.
3 Spoon the mixture into the prepared tins, filling only up to two thirds of the muffin hole. Sprinkle over the remaining oats. Bake for 20 minutes, or until cooked and a skewer inserted into the centre comes out clean.

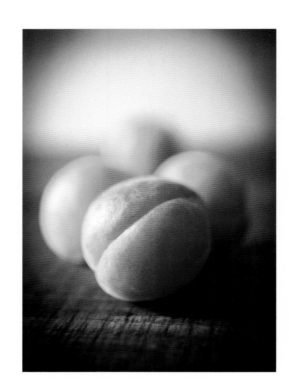

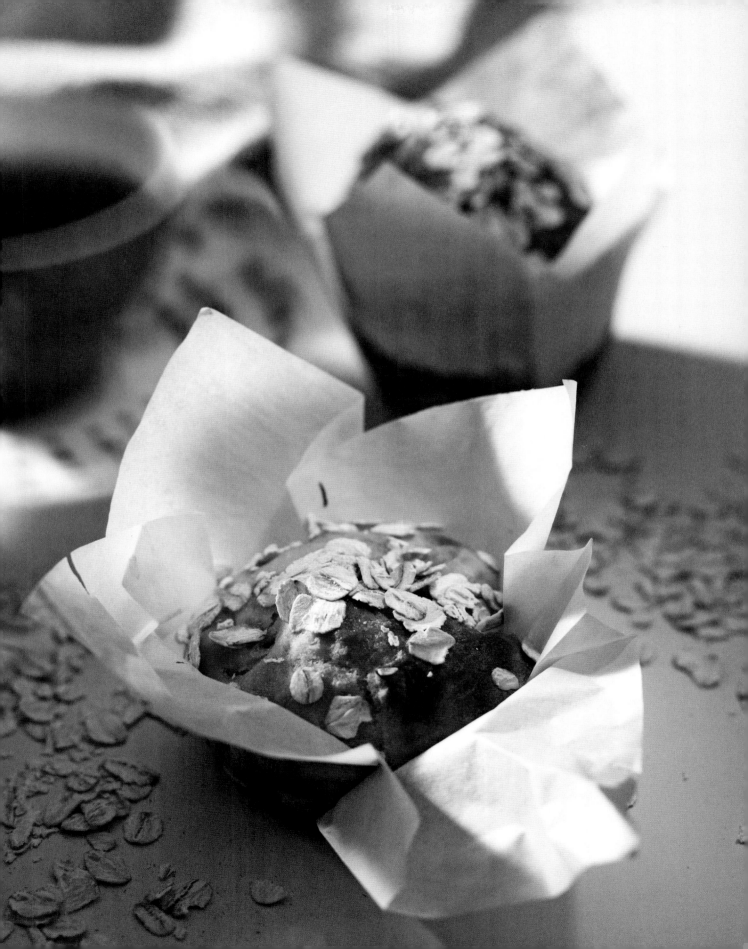

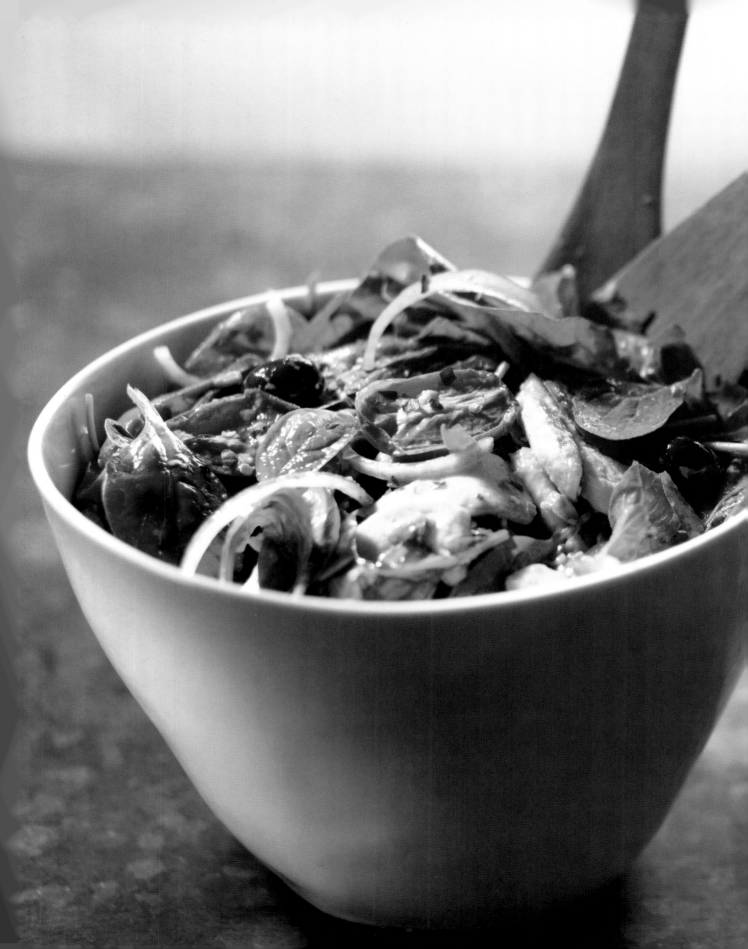

Thank goodness for lunchtime—a chance to stretch your legs, or to sit and enjoy a slice of 'me-time' or 'friends-time' in the middle of the day. Count the benefits of making lunchtime a priority and take the time to refuel, re-energise and socialise.

The food lover's way to a **healthy lunch**

Refuel: Top up your tank with the fuel you need to be at your best for the rest of the day and to power you over the end-of-day finish line.

Re-energise: Recharge your emotional batteries. Taking time out for lunch can help you stay sane and get ahead by making plans for the rest of the day—including the daily question of 'What's for dinner tonight?'

It's good to remember: Lunch is a natural energy shot. A good lunch will provide you with around 15 to 25 counts.

Socialise: Catch up with friends or get to know your work colleagues better. Talking things over, sharing ideas and networking all help you to stay in touch and keep a good perspective on life, and may even open doors to exciting new opportunities.

Q&A

It's good to remember:
A healthy lunch helps you
eat less at dinner.

*Half sandwich made with
1 thick slice of grainy bread
9 counts*

Q: My work day seems to drag on endlessly and some days I hardly have enough energy left to drive myself home. We are a bit short staffed, so I end up skipping lunch if I have to mind the phones, or else I spend my 'break' in front of my computer with something like a juice or smoothie to keep me going. But I am still tired. What should I do?

A: First of all, if you have a full-time job and are working 9 a.m.–5 p.m. (or even longer hours), you really need a lunch break to 're-energise' and 'refuel', as we say. It doesn't have to be a full hour; 20–30 minutes is better than nothing. It's a good idea to go for a brisk walk in the fresh air, making sure to take some deep breaths. It will give your mind and eyes a rest, and it will help you to focus better in the afternoon and be more productive. Take a water bottle to keep hydrated and find a nice spot to eat your lunch. Try a sandwich made with grainy bread and filled with egg, meat, chicken or fish plus salad vegetables, and a piece of fruit instead of large serves of juice or smoothies. Once you get the lunch habit you will find you feel more in control of your day and that the time won't drag.

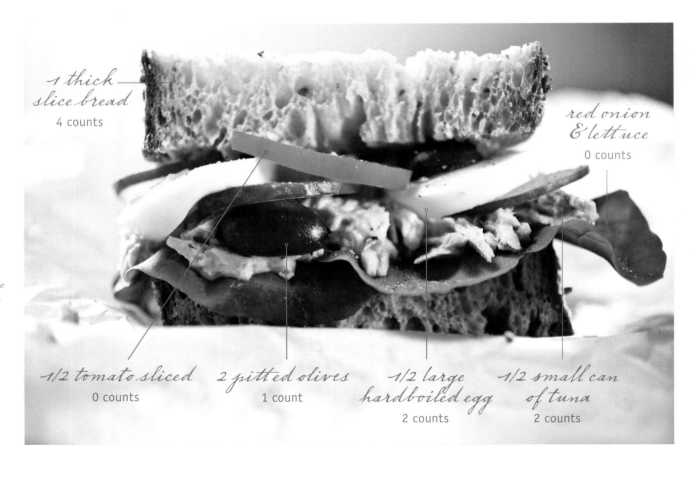

*1 thick
slice bread*
4 counts

*red onion
& lettuce*
0 counts

1/2 tomato sliced
0 counts

2 pitted olives
1 count

*1/2 large
hardboiled egg*
2 counts

*1/2 small can
of tuna*
2 counts

No one else does it

A brisk walk and a bite to eat will make you more productive—whose team members and boss wouldn't want that? If you take the first step, perhaps your colleagues will join you.

I have too much work and I like to leave on time

Use lunchtime as an opportunity to plan the rest of your day (and what's for dinner). It all comes down to smart time management and an achievable 'to do' list.

It's too hot, cold, wet ...

Keep a rain jacket, umbrella, sunscreen, sneakers or running shoes and socks at work, and don't forget a small water bottle in warmer weather.

Make lunch count

Check out the counts for some typical lunches at the sandwich bar, or in the canteen or food hall. Aim for around 15–25 counts at lunchtime most days unless it's your main meal of the day.

14 counts
- Lean mince burger with chilli sauce, tomato, red capsicum, red onion and lettuce on a medium-sized mixed grain roll.
- Greek salad made with tomato, green capsicum, red onion, cucumber, olives, olive oil, lemon juice and feta.
- Medium tub of fresh fruit salad and full-fat plain yoghurt.

15 counts
- Salad sandwich with ham and mustard made with two slices of mixed grain bread, three slices of reduced-salt ham, two teaspoons of reduced-fat mayonnaise, garlic powder, black pepper, lettuce leaves, three thick slices of tomato and one teaspoon of mustard.

17 counts
- Chicken avocado salad made with one quarter of an avocado, one small chicken breast, one tablespoon of chopped red onion, one tablespoon of chopped fresh coriander and 1–2 teaspoons of balsamic vinegar.
- Three fresh (not fried) avocado and chicken rice paper rolls.

Excuse buster

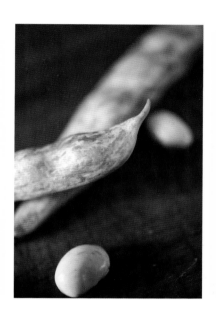

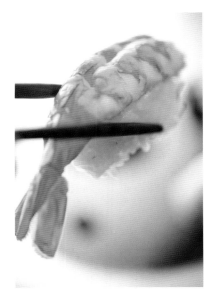

Count to ten with a sushi box of six small pieces.

18 counts

- Curried egg sandwich on wholemeal bread made with two hard-boiled eggs, ½ teaspoon of curry powder, two teaspoons of reduced-fat mayonnaise, shredded lettuce and two slices of mixed grain bread.
- A chicken pasta salad made with half a chicken breast, ½ cup of cooked pasta, one quarter of a red capsicum, one quarter of a green capsicum, five cherry tomatoes and 1 tablespoon of feta cheese, topped with 1 tablespoon of Caesar dressing.

19 counts

- Avocado sandwich made with one third of an avocado, half a sliced tomato, 1 tablespoon of reduced-fat mayonnaise and two slices of mixed grain bread.
- A bowl of thick lentil soup plus a medium-sized grainy roll spread with margarine.

20 counts

- Roast beef and horseradish cream wrap made with one wholemeal wrap, two slices of roast beef, 2 teaspoons of horseradish cream and a handful of lettuce or baby spinach, with a 200g tub of low-fat yoghurt.
- Tuna and avocado roll made with one medium-sized mixed grain roll, a small can of tuna in spring water, one quarter of a medium avocado, two slices of tomato and snipped fresh chives, plus a medium orange.
- Easy bean salad made with ½ cup of four-bean mix, half a chopped celery stalk, one quarter of a red capsicum, diced, 1 tablespoon of mayonnaise and chopped fresh parsley, plus one small glass (¾ cup) orange juice.

21 counts

- Smoked salmon and rocket on toast made with two slices of toasted wholegrain bread, 4 tablespoons of cottage cheese, two slices of smoked salmon, one handful of rocket leaves (and a few capers for extra flavour, if you wish), plus a banana.

23 counts

- Falafel pocket made with one wholemeal pita pocket (or piece of Lebanese bread), two falafel balls cut into half, five slices of cucumber, 1 tablespoon of hummus and 1 tablespoon of full-fat plain yoghurt.

- Packet soup with croutons or noodles—plain or wholegrain—like COUNTRY CUP. Just add boiling water = 5–7 counts. (There are gluten-free options.) Make it a complete meal with a small wholegrain dinner roll spread with 2 tablespoons of low-fat cottage or ricotta cheese = 7 extra counts.
- LEAN CUISINE Bowl range is a great option when you are hungry but short on time. They heat in the microwave in 5–10 minutes = 11–21 counts.
- 2 Minute Noodles—for example, the MAGGI 99% fat free range is baked, not fried, so you save on counts = 15 counts.

Build a better salad

The salad bar has all the makings of a healthy lunch, and there are so many delicious and healthy options. However, don't be seduced by the tempting toppings (like crunchy croutons and crispy bacon bits) and creamy dressings. Our salad bar survival guide will show you how you can build a better salad and feel the difference.

Priority # 1: Eat vegetables

This is one place where you can (almost) throw portion to the wind. We want you to have two cups of salad vegetables—it helps you achieve your five serves of vegetables a day. Check out the most popular salad vegetable options on page 79.

Priority # 2: Go for variety

Go for colour and variety with your salad vegetables and pack in those protective antioxidants—nature's personal bodyguards.

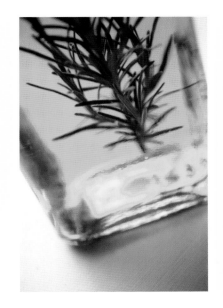

Priority # 3: Dress with care—pick the good fats or low-fat dressings

Be well dressed. Look for low counts or good oils such as mono-unsaturated or polyunsaturated oils like olive, peanut and canola oils.

Priority # 4: Find flavour without salt

Hold the salt shaker and add extra flavour with herbs like basil, mint, parsley or coriander, and aromatics like chopped shallots (spring onions), condiments like Dijon mustard, and, of course, flavoured vinegars like balsamic or raspberry.

The fats of the matter

When choosing oil for cooking or for salad dressings, look for types that are high in mono-unsaturated or polyunsaturated fats, or are a source of omega-3.

- ✔ Mono-unsaturated oils—avocado, olive, canola, peanut, Sunola, macadamia and mustard seed oils.
- ✔ Polyunsaturated oils—safflower, sunflower, grapeseed, soybean, corn, linseed (flaxseed), cottonseed, walnut, sesame oils.

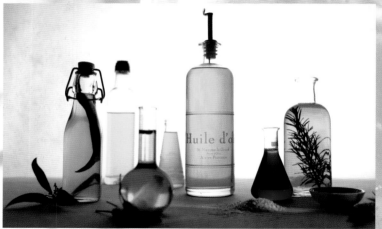

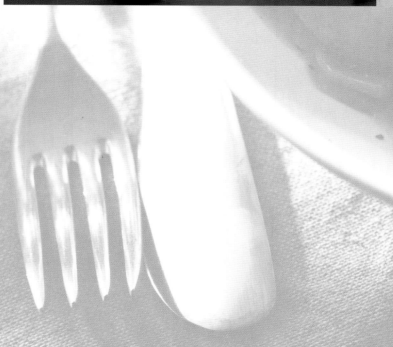

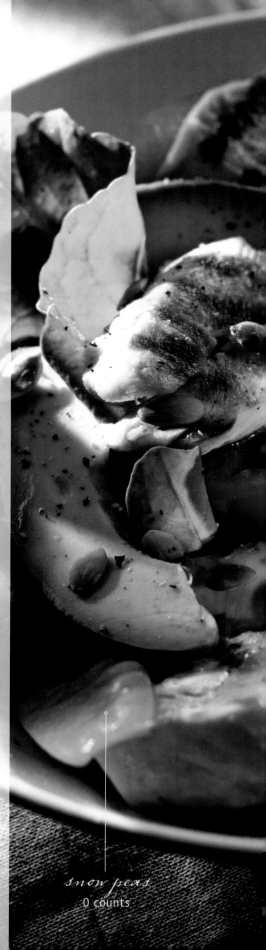

snow peas
0 counts

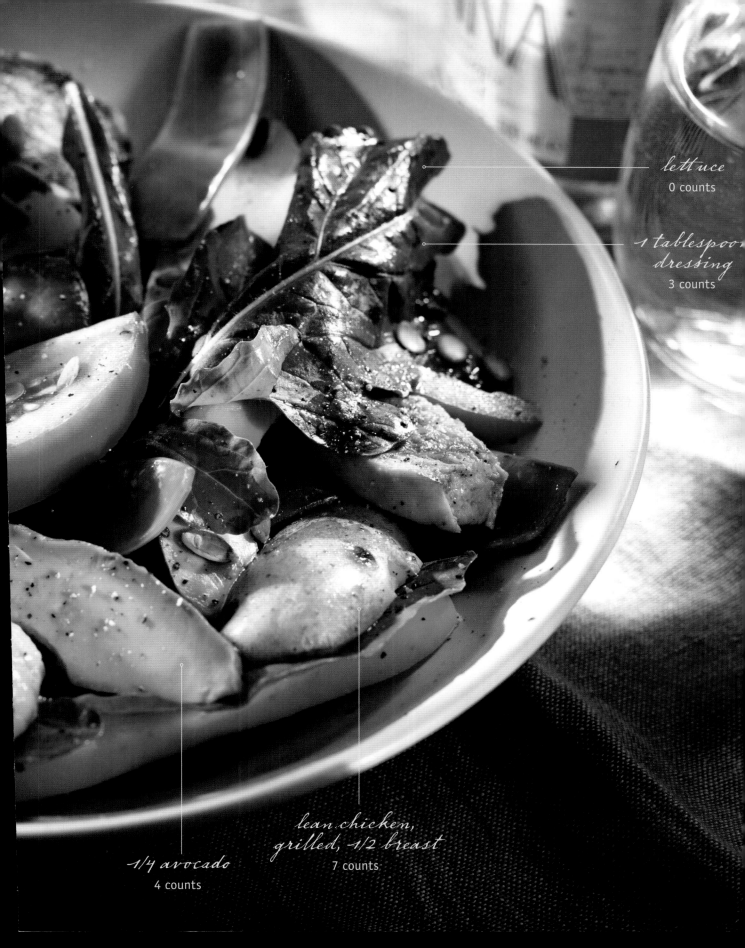

lettuce
0 counts

1 tablespoon
dressing
3 counts

1/4 avocado
4 counts

lean chicken,
grilled, 1/2 breast
7 counts

Size matters

A tub of salad seems like such a healthy option when checking out the canteen or food hall options, but keep an eye on portion size when it contains more than just salad vegetables. Look how the counts add up with small, medium and large salads from 'green' to 'bean', 'pasta' or 'potato', with typical dressings for these salads:

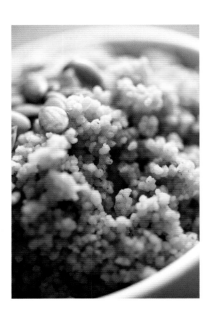

SALAD	SMALL TUB (counts)	MEDIUM TUB (counts)	LARGE TUB (counts)
Garden salad	0	1	2
Coleslaw	12	20	24
Rice salad	13	22	25
Bean salad	13	23	27
Chickpea and pumpkin salad	14	24	28
Lentil and couscous salad	14	24	29
Caesar salad	19	32	38
Potato salad with mayonnaise	21	36	43
Pesto pasta salad	25	42	50

Mix and match your lunch

To refuel and re-energise at lunchtime, choose foods from each of the following food groups:

- Breads, grains and starchy vegetables.
- Meat, chicken, fish, eggs, dairy foods, nuts, seeds and legumes.
- Salad vegetables.
- Fruit.

For most of us, a satisfying lunch will have around 20 counts. The counts we give here are only average counts for these typical foods. Check out the counts for your favourite foods and brands in our ready-reckoner (page 222).

Typical counts for breads, grains and starchy vegetables
- **1 count** = one thin rice cake.
- **2 counts** = one thick rice cake.
- **3 counts** = one medium cob corn.
- **4 counts** = one small (dinner) wholegrain roll; one small (30g) bagel; one small (25g) tortilla; one small pita pocket bread; two sunflower seed and oat crispbreads.
- **5 counts** = one thick slice of grainy wholemeal seed or rye bread; ½ cup of cooked brown or white rice; one medium baked potato in its jacket.
- **6 counts** = two thin slices of wholemeal sandwich bread; quarter of a large (180g) roll of Turkish bread (pide).
- **7 counts** = one medium wholegrain 'dinner' roll; one small piece of focaccia; one medium wholemeal pita (pocket bread); one wholemeal English muffin; one small wholemeal wrap; four crispy rye crackers; ½ cup of cooked pasta; three small pieces of sushi.
- **9 counts** = two slices of dense grainy bread.
- **10 counts** = one small (90g) wholegrain long roll.
- **11 counts** = ½ cup of cooked rice noodles.
- **19 counts** = one large (170g) wholegrain long roll.

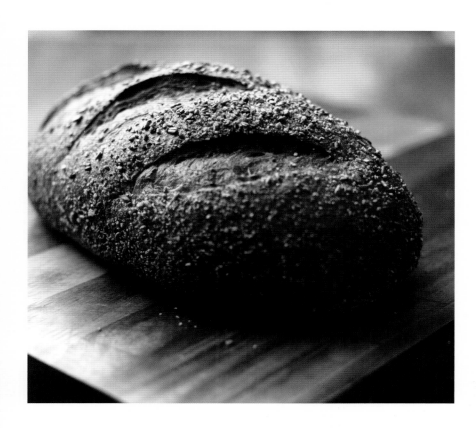

1/2 cup lentils
5 counts

celery sticks
0 counts

tuna
4 counts

1 small
slice salmon
1 count

1 large egg
4 counts

2 slices of ham
6 counts

Typical counts for meat, chicken, fish, eggs, dairy foods, nuts and legumes

- **1 count =** 1 tablespoon of cottage cheese or ricotta; one slice of smoked salmon.
- **2 counts =** ½ cup of reduced-fat or skim milk.
- **3 counts =** one medium (47g) hard-boiled egg; ten almonds; 1 tablespoon of sunflower seeds; two thin slices of deli roast beef; one regular slice of lean leg ham (off the bone) or two thin slices of lean (97% fat free) packaged ham.
- **4 counts =** 200g tub of diet yoghurt; one small (95g) can of tuna or salmon in spring water (drained); one large hard-boiled egg; four thin slices of pastrami.
- **5 counts =** one slice of reduced-fat cheddar cheese; ½ cup of cooked tofu; ½ cup of cooked or canned beans, chickpeas or lentils; two small (6cm) falafel patties; 1 cup of packet pea-and-ham soup (from one sachet).
- **6 counts =** ½ cup of baked beans in tomato sauce; 105g can of pink salmon in spring water (drained).
- **7 counts =** two cheese sticks; six thin deli slices of lean ham; four thin deli slices of trimmed turkey or three deli slices of chicken breast.
- **8 counts =** 1 cup of bean salad.

Typical counts for salad vegetables

Enjoy countless quantities of salad vegetables—just watch the dressing and toppings (see fats and oils).

- **Free =** loose-leaf lettuce leaves (mesclun mix); rocket; baby spinach; coleslaw; Asian greens; onion rings; shallots (spring onions); sliced mushrooms; sliced cucumber; grated/shredded/shaved carrot; capsicum slices; celery sticks; tiny tomatoes; radishes; sprouts; herbs; crunchy beans; snow peas; blanched broccoli; canned beetroot slices; canned asparagus spears; fresh tomato salsa; jarred artichokes (in brine).

It's good to remember:
Most dips will be 2–3 counts
per tablespoon.

Typical counts for fats and oils

- **1 count** = 1 teaspoon of pesto; 2 teaspoons of fat-free salad dressings; 1 tablespoon of 97% fat-free mayonnaise; 1 tablespoon of mashed or one slice of avocado; 1 tablespoon of extra-light cream cheese.
- **2 counts** = 1 teaspoon of olive oil; 1 teaspoon of margarine or butter; 1 tablespoon of light cream cheese; 1 tablespoon of honey mustard dressing; 1 tablespoon of hummus.
- **3 counts** = ½ tablespoon of hollandaise sauce; 1 tablespoon of full-fat cream cheese; 1 tablespoon of pesto.
- **4 counts** = 2 teaspoons of regular mayonnaise; 2 tablespoons of pesto.
- **5 counts** = one half of a small avocado.
- **7 counts** = 1 tablespoon of traditional mayonnaise.

Typical counts for condiments

- **1 count** = 2 teaspoons of grainy mustard; 2 teaspoons of horseradish cream; 1 tablespoon of tomato sauce; 1 tablespoon of BRANSTON pickles.
- **2 counts** = 1 tablespoon of sweet chilli sauce; 1 tablespoon of fruit chutney.
- **3 counts** = 2 tablespoons of cranberry jelly.

Typical counts for fruit

- **2 counts** = one medium mandarin; half a medium pawpaw (or papaya); two large apricots; ½ cup of blueberries.
- **3 counts** = one medium kiwifruit; one large peach or nectarine; two medium plums; 1 cup of pineapple cubes; one (3cm) thick slice of watermelon.
- **4 counts** = 1 cup of fresh fruit salad; one medium apple; one small banana; one medium orange; one medium pear; half a rockmelon; small bunch (22) grapes; ½ cup of canned fruit (in juice or water); one small glass (200ml/ ¾ cup) orange, apple or mango juice.
- **5 counts** = one small glass (200ml/¾ cup) pomegranate juice.

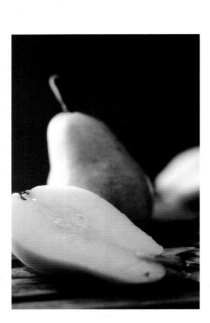

You'll save counts if you have a piece of fruit and water with your lunch instead of a bottle of juice.

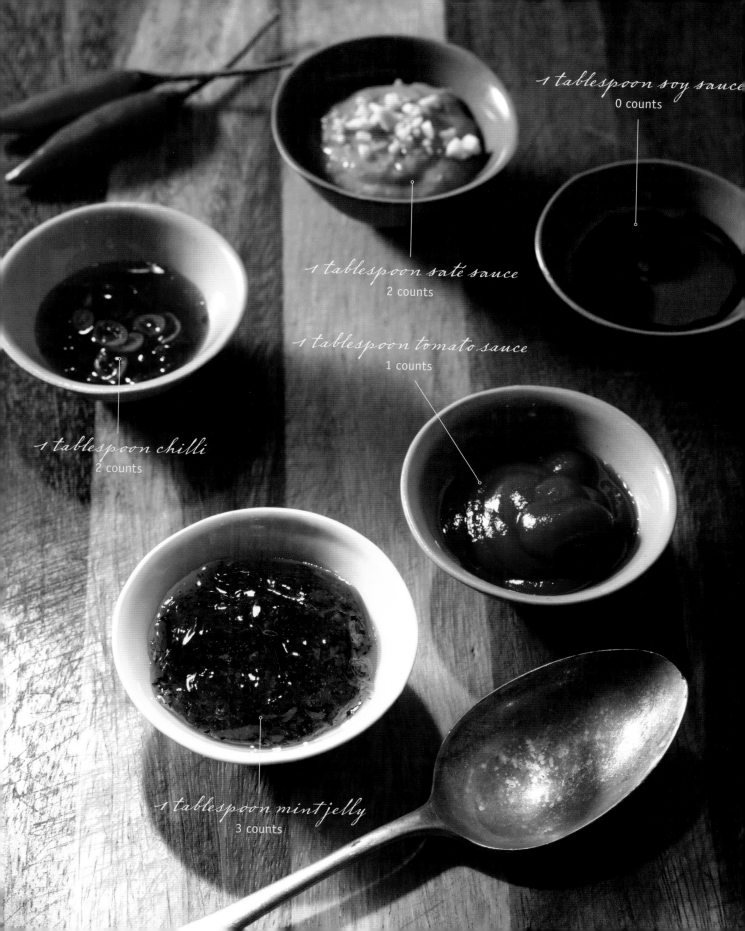

1 tablespoon soy sauce
0 counts

1 tablespoon saté sauce
2 counts

1 tablespoon tomato sauce
1 counts

1 tablespoon chilli
2 counts

1 tablespoon mint jelly
3 counts

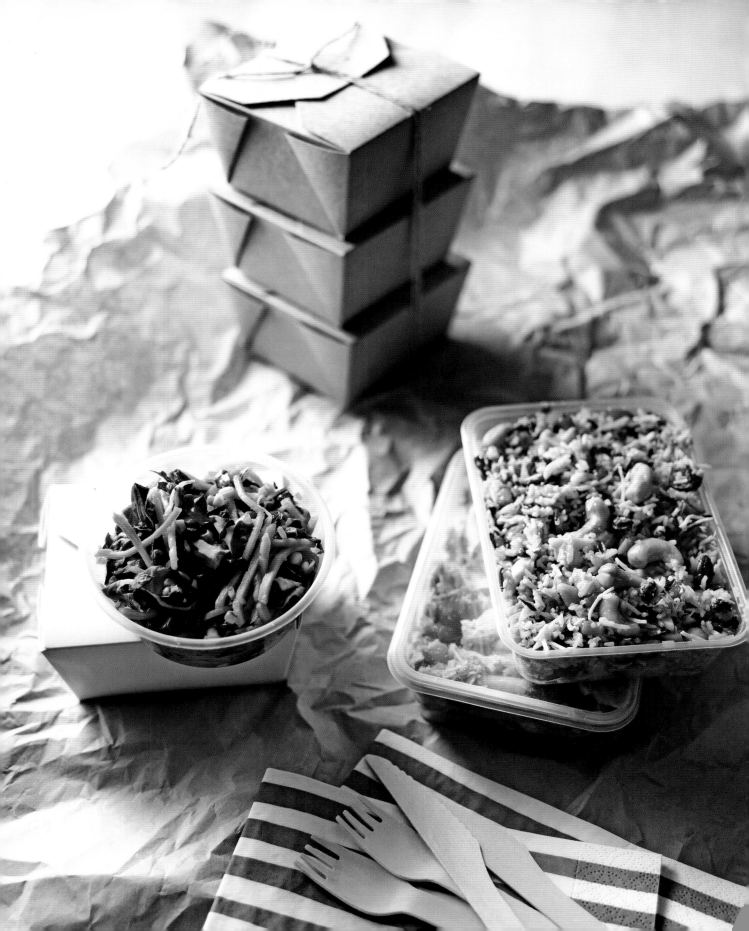

How to save counts eating out and choosing takeaways

When eating out or ordering a takeaway, remember to run your eyes carefully over the menu. Count the difference and choose wisely.

CHOOSE THIS	NOT THAT
1 cup of steamed rice = 9 counts	1 cup of fried rice = 17 counts
1 medium bowl of chicken and corn soup = 8 counts	1 medium bowl of seafood laksa = 13 counts
1 fresh rice paper roll = 4 counts	1 deep-fried spring roll = 19 counts
1 small piece of grilled fish without batter = 5 counts	1 small piece of deep-fried crumbed fish = 10 counts
1 medium bowl of spaghetti bolognaise = 14 counts	1 medium bowl of spaghetti carbonara = 23 counts
1 taco with meat, cheese and salad = 12 counts	1 cup of nachos with sour cream = 18 counts
1 steak and salad sandwich with 1 lean piece of minute steak, tomato, lettuce, cucumber, grated carrot and mayonnaise = 19 counts	1 fried schnitzel sandwich with creamy coleslaw = 24 counts
1 medium jacket potato = 7 counts	1 regular serving of hot chips = 22 counts
2 slices of roast lamb with 1 baked potato, vegetables and gravy = 17 counts	Steak sandwich made with 2 slices of white sandwich bread, with fried steak, fried onions, lettuce, tomato and sauce = 27 counts
1 cup of Greek salad = 14 counts	1 cup of chicken caesar salad = 18 counts
2 slices of thin and crispy vegetable pizza = 13 counts	2 slices of cheese crust pizza with peperoni = 23 counts
Small bowl dhal = 6 counts	1 samosa = 25 counts
3 cheese and spinach triangles (filo pastry) = 10 counts	Beef, mushroom and onion pie = 20 counts
¼ roasted chicken without skin = 9 counts	¼ roasted chicken with skin = 13 counts
1 regular hot dog (medium roll and sausage) = 18 counts	1 regular cheeseburger with fried beef pattie, 1 slice of light cheese, onion, tomato sauce and margarine = 25 counts
1 medium serve of chicken tikka = 13 counts	1 medium serve of butter chicken = 22 counts

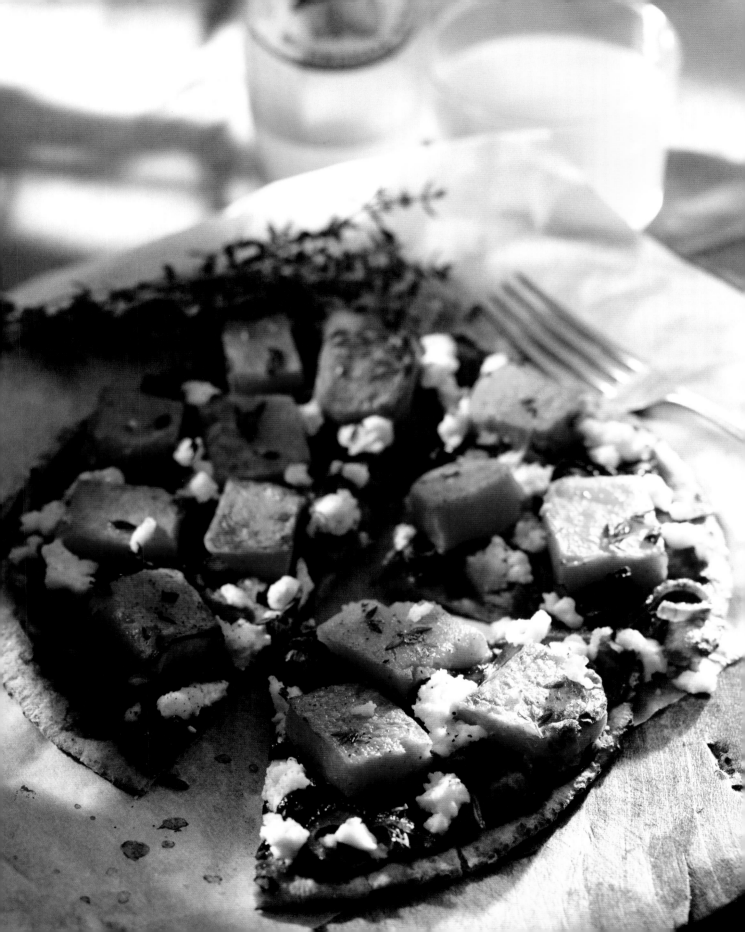

Healthy lunch recipes

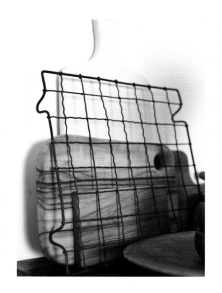

Roasted pumpkin and ricotta pita pizza

250g pumpkin, deseeded, peeled and cut into 3cm pieces

olive or canola oil spray

½ tsp dried oregano, or to taste

freshly ground black pepper

1 wholemeal pita

2 tbsp tomato paste

baby spinach leaves

½ red onion, thinly sliced

¼ cup fresh ricotta, lightly crumbled

1 cup rocket leaves, to serve

1 Preheat the oven to 200°C (180°C fan-forced). Line a baking tray with baking paper.
2 Place the pumpkin pieces in an ovenproof baking dish and lightly spray with oil, making sure they are evenly coated. Sprinkle over the oregano and season with pepper. Bake for 25 minutes, or until tender. Remove from the oven.
3 Place the pita bread on the prepared baking tray and spread evenly with the tomato paste. Top with pumpkin pieces, baby spinach and onion. Scatter over the ricotta. Bake for 10 minutes or until the base is crisp.
4 Serve topped with rocket leaves.

PREP: 10 mins
COOK: 35 mins
SERVES: 2
COUNTS PER SERVE: 15

KEEP COUNT OF PIZZA TOPPINGS
Vegetables and fruit counts
¼ CUP CHOPPED OLIVES: 2
½ CUP DICED PINEAPPLE: 2
¼ MEDIUM AVOCADO: 4
Cheese counts
¼ CUP GRATED LOW-FAT CHEDDAR: 6
¼ CUP LOW-FAT FETA, CRUMBLED: 7
¼ CUP FRESH RICOTTA, CRUMBLED: 5
Meat, chicken and seafood counts
70G BEEF OR LAMB STRIPS: 6
70G SKINLESS COOKED CHICKEN
  BREAST: 6
50G SALAMI SLICES: 10
50G LEAN DICED HAM: 3
½ CUP COOKED PRAWNS: 4

Creamy parsnip and cauliflower soup

Save the cauliflower florets to serve as a vegetable side dish and use the sweet stem that's often thrown away in this nourishing and economical soup. To make this a vegetarian meal, use vegetable stock instead of chicken.

PREP: 10 mins
COOK: 15 mins
SERVES: 6
COUNTS PER SERVE: 9

1 tsp olive or canola oil

1 medium onion, chopped

4 large parsnips, peeled and chopped or sliced into rounds

1 large potato, peeled and chopped or diced

1 cup chopped cauliflower stem

2 cups chicken stock

375ml CARNATION Light & Creamy Evaporated Milk

¼ cup roughly chopped walnuts

1 Heat the oil in a large saucepan and cook the onion for 2 minutes, or until just soft. Add parsnips, potatoes, cauliflower and stock. Bring to the boil, then reduce the heat to low and simmer, covered, for 12 minutes or until the vegetables are soft.
2 Remove the pan from the heat, add the evaporated milk and, when cool, blend to a creamy puree.
3 Gently reheat (don't let it boil) and serve sprinkled with walnuts.

Barley and vegetable soup

Barley is great stick-to-the-ribs food when feeding a hungry family. It's also very versatile—it can do anything rice can do, but is all too often left on the pantry shelf because it takes a bit longer to cook. We have used it in a traditional barley and vegetable soup here, but it makes a wonderful risotto and is delicious added to casseroles for one-dish dinners.

PREP: 15 mins
COOK: 40 mins
SERVES: 4
COUNTS PER SERVE: 8

1 tsp olive oil

1 medium onion, chopped

1 medium carrot, diced

400g can tomatoes

1 tbsp tomato paste

½ cup pearl barley

4 cups vegetable stock

1 cup fresh or frozen peas

100g baby spinach leaves

2 tbsp roughly chopped fresh herbs (e.g., parsley, basil and oregano)

freshly ground black pepper, to taste

1 Heat the oil in a heavy-based saucepan, add the onion and cook, covered, over low heat for about 5 minutes, or until the onion is soft. Add the carrots, tomatoes, tomato paste, barley and prepared stock. Bring to the boil, reduce the heat to low and simmer for 30 minutes.
2 Stir in the peas and simmer for 2–3 minutes, then add the spinach and herbs, and simmer for a further 1–2 minutes until heated through and the barley is cooked.
3 Ladle the soup into four bowls, season with pepper and serve.

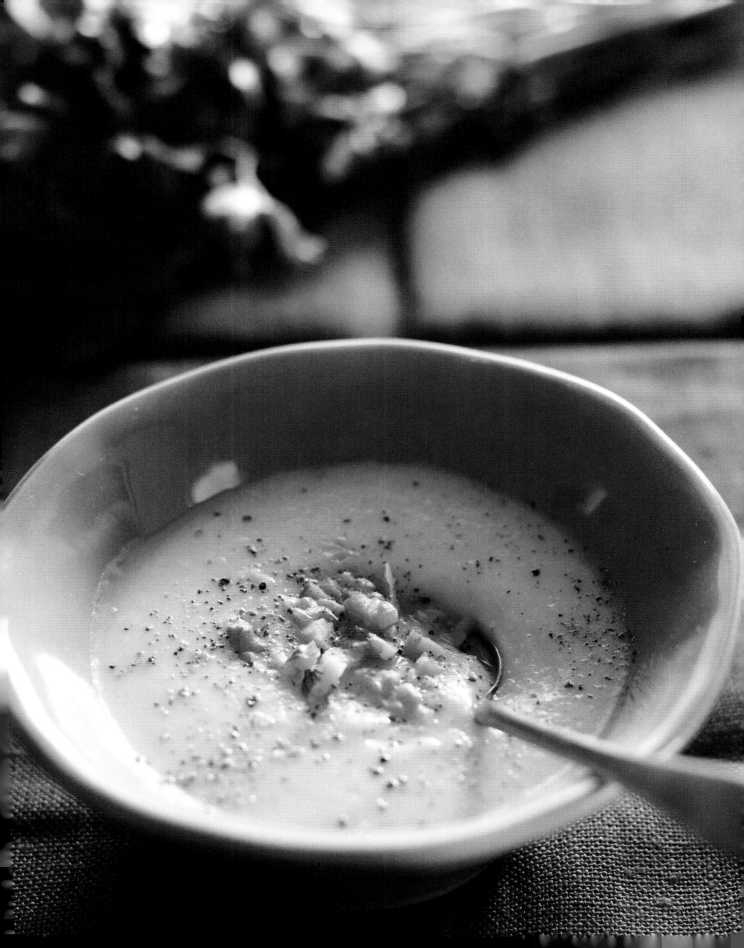

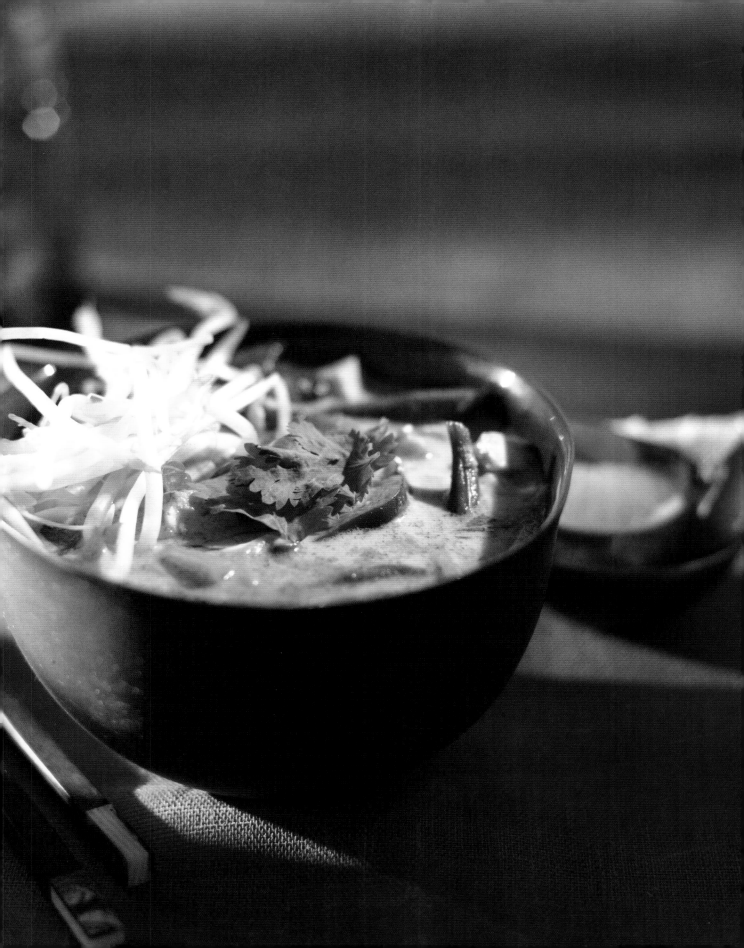

Vegetarian laksa

125g dried rice-stick noodles

⅓ cup red curry paste

300g firm tofu cut into 1cm cubes

2 cups chicken stock

1 small eggplant, chopped coarsley

100g fresh shiitake mushrooms, thinly sliced

125g green beans, diagonally sliced

3 baby bok choy, separated, washed and shredded

1 tbsp brown sugar

375ml CARNATION Light & Creamy Coconut Flavoured Evaporated Milk

65g bean sprouts

½ cup picked coriander leaves

lime wedges to serve

This laksa is made using coconut-flavoured evaporated milk instead of coconut milk, so you can enjoy a laksa with less fat and more protein and calcium. Add a dash of chilli if you want to turn up the heat.

PREP: 15 mins
COOK: 10 mins
SERVES: 4
COUNTS PER SERVE: 17

1 Cook the noodles in a large saucepan of boiling water for 2 minutes, or until just tender. Drain well and divide among four large bowls.

2 Heat a large wok over high heat, add the curry paste, eggplant and tofu, and cook for 2 minutes. Add the stock, mushrooms and beans, and cook for another 2 minutes. Add the bok choy and cook for a further minute, or until tender. Add the sugar and coconut-flavoured evaporated milk, then bring to a simmer.

3 Pour the liquid evenly into the bowls, top with the bean sprouts and coriander, and serve with lime wedges if desired.

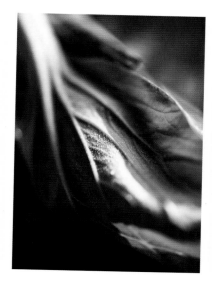

A pastry brush is handy for brushing the chilli sauce over the sweet potato chunks to make sure the flavour is evenly spread. You can also make this salad with pumpkin chunks, but you would need to reduce the baking time. We love this tangy recipe because it's a complete meal in itself, and by using a diet yoghurt you can keep the creamy dressing counts down while boosting your calcium and protein intake.

PREP: 10 mins
COOK: 40 mins
SERVES: 4
COUNTS PER SERVE: 11

Sweet potato and chickpea salad

1kg orange-fleshed sweet potato, peeled and cut into large chunks

1½ tbsp sweet chilli sauce

4 shallots (spring onions), sliced

100g baby spinach leaves

¼ cup pepitas (pumpkin seeds)

420g can chickpeas, rinsed and drained

juice from half a medium lemon

400g diet natural yoghurt

1 cup chopped fresh coriander leaves

1 Preheat the oven to 200°C (180°C fan-forced).
2 Place the sweet potato on a non-stick baking tray and drizzle over the sweet chilli sauce. Bake for 40 minutes, or until the sweet potato is caramelised and soft, turning once during the cooking time. Allow to cool.
3 Transfer the sweet potato to a large serving bowl and add shallots, baby spinach, pepitas and chickpeas. Gently toss together to combine.
4 To make the dressing, whisk together the lemon juice, yoghurt and coriander. Drizzle over the salad and serve immediately.

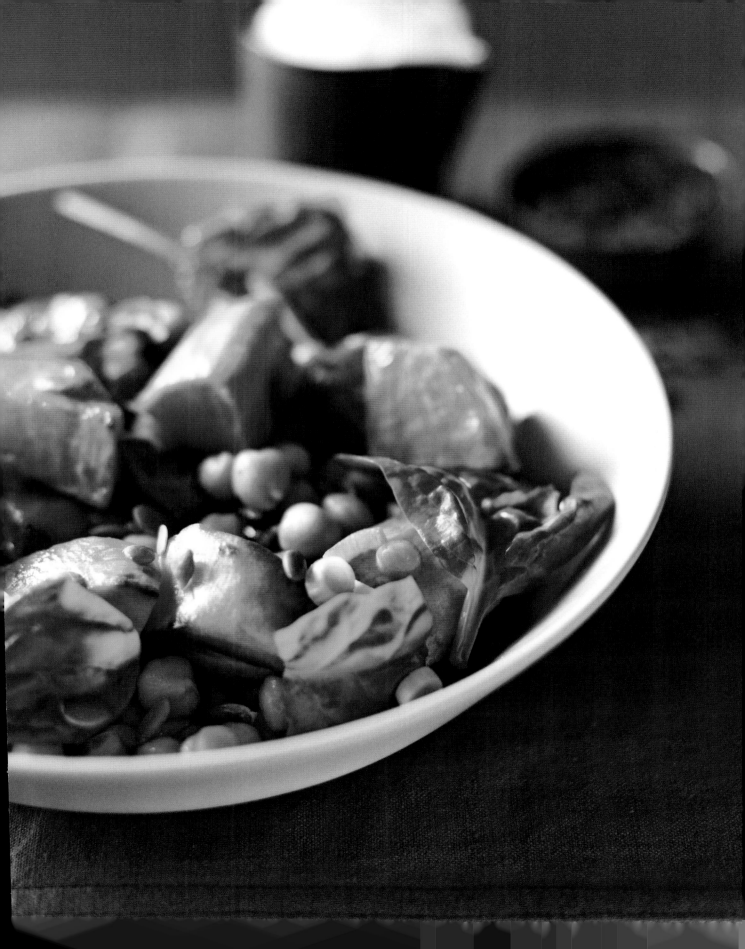

Mirin has been used in Japanese cooking for centuries. It is a type of rice wine, and can usually be found in the supermarket alongside other Asian cooking ingredients like soy sauce and miso. It's extremely versatile—use it in Asian vegetable slaw, miso soup, Asian salad dressings, sushi and sushi dipping sauces, or simply add a tablespoon or two to the water when steaming or boiling vegetables or rice.

PREP: 20 mins
COOK: 10 mins
SERVES: 4
COUNTS PER SERVE: 14

Soba noodle soup with prawns and tofu

100g soba noodles

4 cups vegetable stock

2 tsp grated fresh ginger

2 tbsp soy sauce

1 tbsp mirin

2 tsp caster sugar

2 small red chillies, seeded and finely chopped

24 raw prawns, peeled and deveined with tails intact

2 shallots (spring onions), sliced on the diagonal

50g baby spinach leaves, shredded

300g silken or firm tofu, cut into 2cm cubes

2 tbsp chopped fresh coriander leaves

1 Cook the soba noodles according to the packet instructions. Drain and set aside.
2 Combine the stock, ginger, soy sauce, mirin, sugar and chillies in a large saucepan. Bring to the boil, then reduce the heat and simmer for 3 minutes. Add the prawns, shallots and spinach, and simmer for 2 minutes, or until the prawns turn pink and are cooked.
3 Divide the noodles and tofu evenly among four bowls. Ladle over the soup and serve topped with fresh coriander leaves.

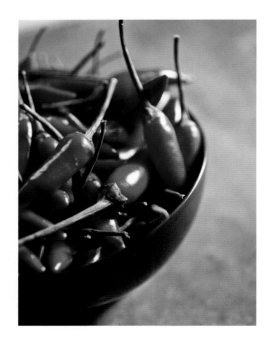

Potato, spinach and mushroom frittata

1 tbsp canola or olive oil

2 medium potatoes, peeled and thinly sliced

1 cup sliced button mushrooms

1 clove garlic, crushed

100g baby spinach leaves

¼ cup chopped shallots (spring onions)

1 tsp chicken stock powder

6 large eggs, lightly beaten

½ cup grated tasty cheese

small bunch parsley, leaves finely chopped (optional)

This frittata makes a very satisfying lunch or light meal. Make sure you use a pan that you can safely pop under a hot grill.

PREP: 10 mins
COOK: 12 mins
SERVES: 6
COUNTS PER SERVE: 10

1 Heat 2 teaspoons of the oil in a large frying pan. Arrange the potato slices evenly over the base of the pan in a single layer, and cover and cook over a gentle heat for 5 minutes. Turn the slices over, then cover and cook for a further 2 minutes, or until tender. Remove the potatoes from the pan and set aside, keeping them warm.

2 Preheat the grill to high. Add the remaining oil, mushrooms and garlic to the pan and cook for 1 minute. Gently stir through the potatoes, spinach, shallots and stock powder. Pour over the beaten eggs and cook over a low heat until the underside of the frittata is golden brown.

3 Sprinkle the cheese evenly over the top and place the pan under a preheated grill until the egg is set—don't let the cheese burn. Cut into wedges and serve sprinkled with the fresh parsley if desired.

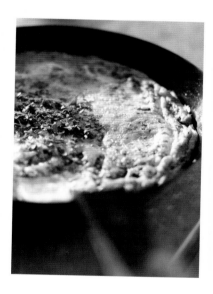

PREP: 10 mins
COOK: 15 mins
SERVES: 4
COUNTS PER SERVE: 15

Thai chicken salad

375ml CARNATION Light & Creamy Coconut Flavoured Evaporated Milk

1 tsp grated fresh ginger

400g chicken breast fillet, thinly sliced

125g rice vermicelli noodles

1 Spanish (red) onion, thinly sliced

1 Lebanese cucumber, cut into thin batons

1 carrot, cut into thin batons

1 tbsp hot chilli sauce

2 tsp fish sauce

1 tsp lime zest

1 cup roughly chopped coriander

1 cup roughly chopped fresh mint leaves

1 tbsp crushed unsalted peanuts

1 Bring the coconut-flavoured evaporated milk and ginger just to the boil in a large frying pan. Reduce the heat and add the chicken, stirring gently to break up the meat. Simmer for 5 minutes, or until cooked through. Lift the chicken out of the pan, place in a dish and set aside.

2 While the chicken is cooking, prepare the vermicelli noodles according to the packet instructions. When the noodles are soft, drain immediately and snip into smaller lengths with kitchen scissors.

3 Add the softened noodles to the frying pan and simmer gently for 5 minutes, until most of the milk has been absorbed. Remove the pan from the heat and let the noodles cool to room temperature.

4 Meanwhile, place the onion, cucumber and carrot in a serving bowl with the hot chilli and fish sauces, and the lime zest. Add the chicken, noodles, coriander, mint and peanuts, then toss so the flavours are well combined and serve.

Chicken, mushroom and broccoli risotto

olive or canola oil spray

400g skinless chicken breast fillets, cut into cubes

1 medium onion, chopped

1½ cups arborio rice

1 packet mushroom soup mix

3¼ cups boiling water

½ cup white wine or water

3 cups broccoli florets

1 cup sliced button mushrooms

2 tsp lemon zest

juice of 1 lemon

¼ cup grated parmesan cheese

freshly ground black pepper

1 tbsp chopped fresh parsley

1 Spray a large non-stick frying pan with oil, and heat. Add the chicken and onion, and cook for 4 minutes over medium heat, stirring. Add the rice and cook, stirring, for another minute. Remove from the heat and stir in the mushroom soup mix.

2 Pour the boiling water and wine carefully into the rice mixture, and return to the heat. Bring to the boil, stirring. Reduce the heat to low, cover and simmer for 15 minutes, stirring occasionally.

3 Stir in the broccoli florets, mushroom slices and lemon zest. Cover and simmer, stirring occasionally, for a further 5 minutes, or until the rice is tender and the liquid absorbed.

4 Stir through the lemon juice and parmesan cheese, and season to taste with freshly ground black pepper. Top with a sprinkling of chopped fresh parsley and serve.

Arborio is a medium-grain rice with a high starch content, and that's what gives risotto dishes their creamy texture. If you just use a regular medium-grain rice, you won't get the same texture, although, of course, the taste will still be great.

PREP: 10 mins
COOK: 30 mins
SERVES: 6
COUNTS PER SERVE: 16

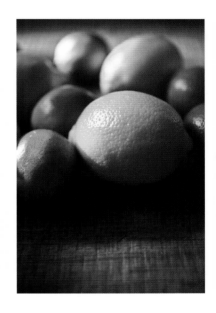

PREP: 20 mins
MAKES: 12
COUNTS PER ROLL: 8

Vietnamese spring rolls

12 x 22cm round rice papers

1 Lebanese cucumber cut into short, thin sticks

1 small red capsicum cut into short, thin strips

1 large carrot, peeled and cut into short, thin sticks

1 small avocado cut into short, thin slices

50g snow pea sprouts, ends trimmed

¾ cup picked coriander leaves

¾ cup picked mint leaves

⅓ cup unsalted roasted peanuts, finely chopped

Dipping sauce

3 tbsp sweet chilli sauce

1½ tbsp soy sauce

3 tbsp fresh lime juice

1 Half-fill a large bowl with warm water. Dip one rice paper in the water for 20 seconds, or until it is just soft. Drain off the excess water and place on a clean surface.

2 Place a few pieces of each of the remaining ingredients on the wrapper, about 3cm from the edge. Fold up the bottom of the wrapper. Fold in the sides and roll up to enclose the filling. Place on a tray and cover with damp paper towels. Repeat with the remaining wrappers and filling ingredients.

3 To make the dipping sauce, combine all sauce ingredients in a bowl.

4 Serve the rice paper rolls with the dipping sauce.

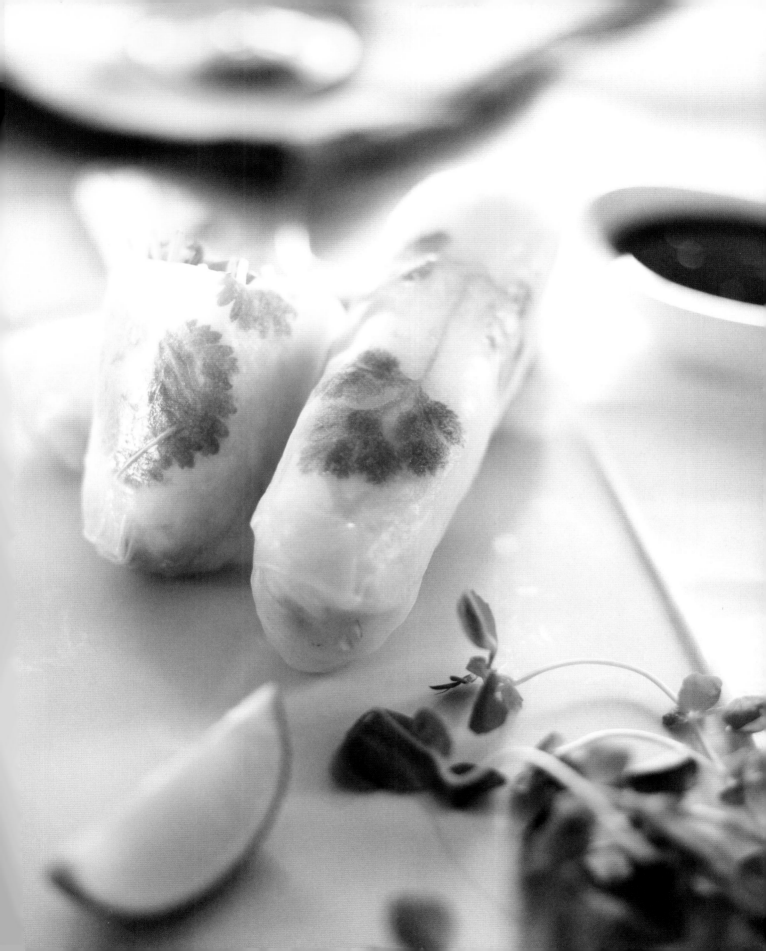

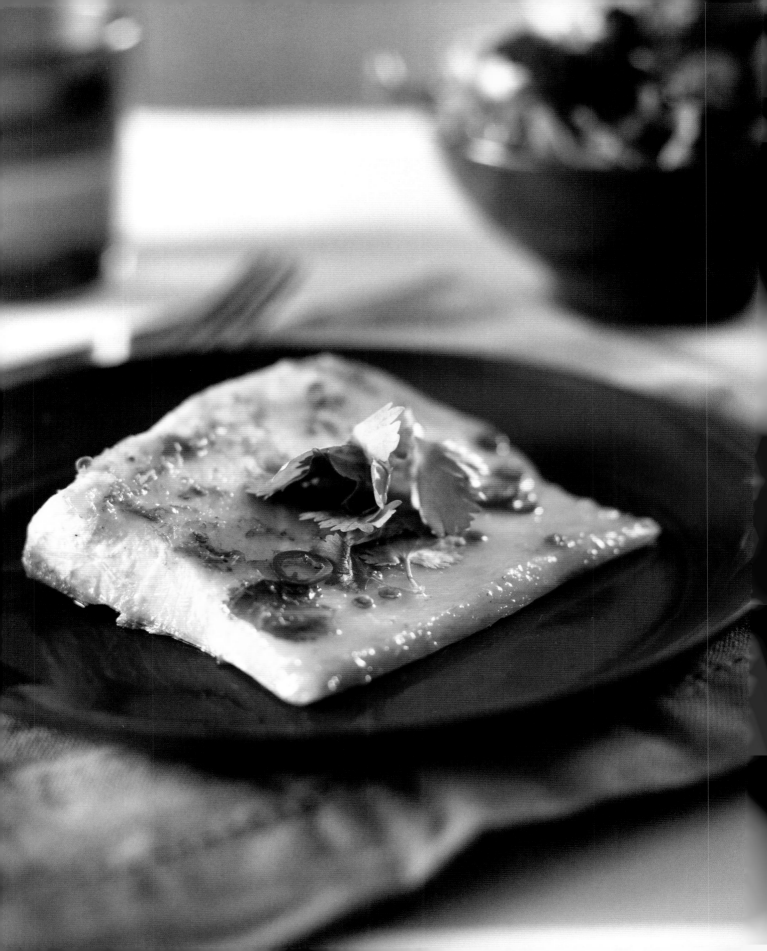

Chilli lime fish

2 tbsp sweet chilli sauce

1 tsp vegetable or garlic stock powder

juice and zest of 1 lime

4 white fish fillets such as sea perch or similar firm-fleshed fish
(about 180g each)

¼ cup chopped fresh coriander leaves

1 Preheat the oven to 200°C (180°C fan-forced).
2 Cut four squares of foil large enough to wrap the fish parcels.
3 Place the sweet chilli sauce, stock powder, lime juice and zest in a
   small bowl or jug, and whisk to combine.
4 Place each fish fillet on a square of foil, evenly drizzle or brush the
   sauce over the fish, sprinkle with coriander leaves and wrap to form
   four individual parcels.
5 Bake in the preheated oven for 10 minutes, or until cooked.

Cooking fish in a parcel in the oven is a great way to cut the counts. You can also barbecue fish in foil this way. Serve this dish with crusty wholegrain bread and a crispy green salad of mixed leaves to make a complete meal.

PREP: 5 mins
COOK: 10 mins
SERVES: 4
COUNTS: 10
SMALL BREAD ROLL: 5 counts

Ten-minute couscous

1½ cups chicken stock

1½ cups couscous

1 medium red capsicum, finely diced

½ cup corn kernels

200g cooked skinless chicken, shredded

2 tbsp chopped fresh parsley

1 Bring the stock to the boil in a medium saucepan.
2 Stir in the couscous using a fork—this prevents the fragile grains
   from squashing, resulting in lumpy couscous—then add the
   remaining ingredients. Remove from the heat, cover and stand for
   5 minutes.
3 Fluff up with the fork and serve.

We prefer to use frozen corn kernels for this recipe as they are quick and easy, and have a better flavour than canned kernels. Of course, when corn is in season there's nothing more delicious than kernels straight from the cob. This recipe is a great way to use up leftover chicken. If you make it with a barbecue chicken, make sure you remove the skin.

PREP: 4 mins
COOK: 1 min
STAND: 5 mins
SERVES: 4
COUNTS PER SERVE: 16

Beef curry

This is an ideal wintery weekend lunch dish for when people are coming home from morning sport, or are off to watch a match in the afternoon. It's a tasty curry, not a hot one. We make our own spice mix in this recipe, but you can use your favourite curry powder if you prefer and add a dash of chilli if you like it hotter.

PREP: 10 mins
COOK: 40 mins
SERVES: 6
COUNTS PER SERVE: 18
COUNTS WITHOUT RICE: 9

olive or canola oil spray

1 medium onion, chopped

1 tsp ground coriander

2 tsp ground cumin

2 tsp ground turmeric

1 tsp crushed garlic

500g lean beef, cut into 2–3cm cubes

400g can crushed tomatoes

1 cup beef stock

1 medium zucchini, sliced

1 cup peeled and diced orange-fleshed sweet potato

150g green beans, cut into 4cm lengths

1½ cups basmati rice

2 tbsp chopped fresh coriander, optional

1 Spray a non-stick pan with oil, and cook the onion, spices and garlic over medium heat for 2–3 minutes, or until the onion is soft. Add the beef and cook for 3–5 minutes, or until browned on all sides. Add the tomatoes and stock, reduce the heat to low and simmer, covered, for 10 minutes. Add the zucchini and sweet potato, and simmer for a further 15 minutes, or until the meat is tender and the vegetables are cooked. Add the beans and cook for another 5 minutes.

2 While the curry is cooking, prepare the rice according to the packet instructions.

3 Sprinkle the chopped fresh coriander over the curry and serve with a scoop of rice.

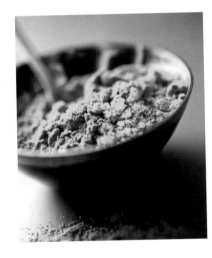

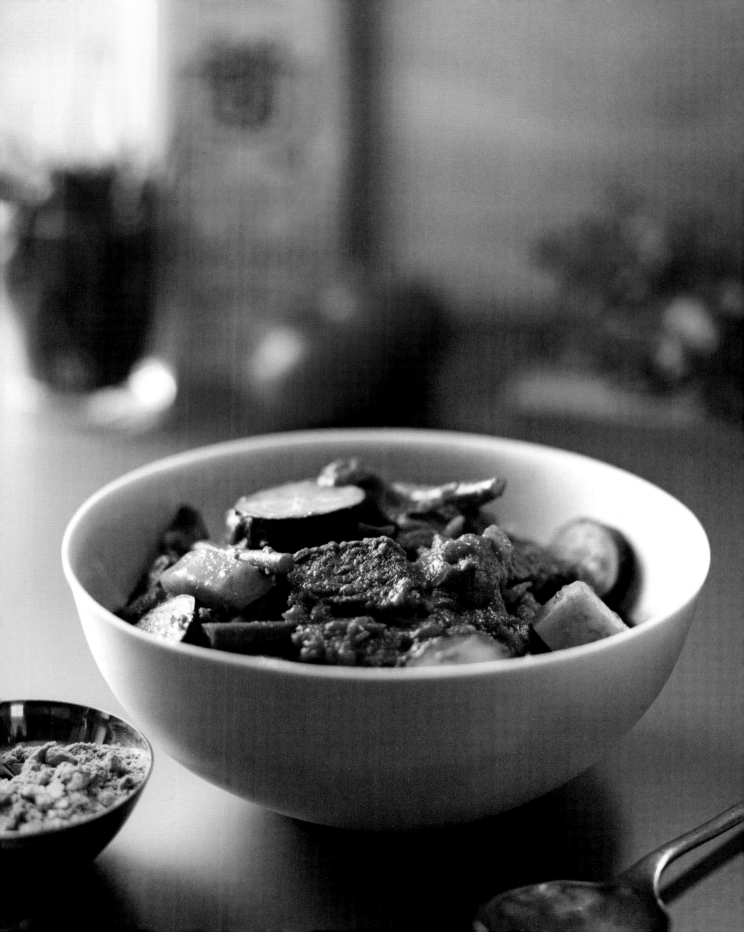

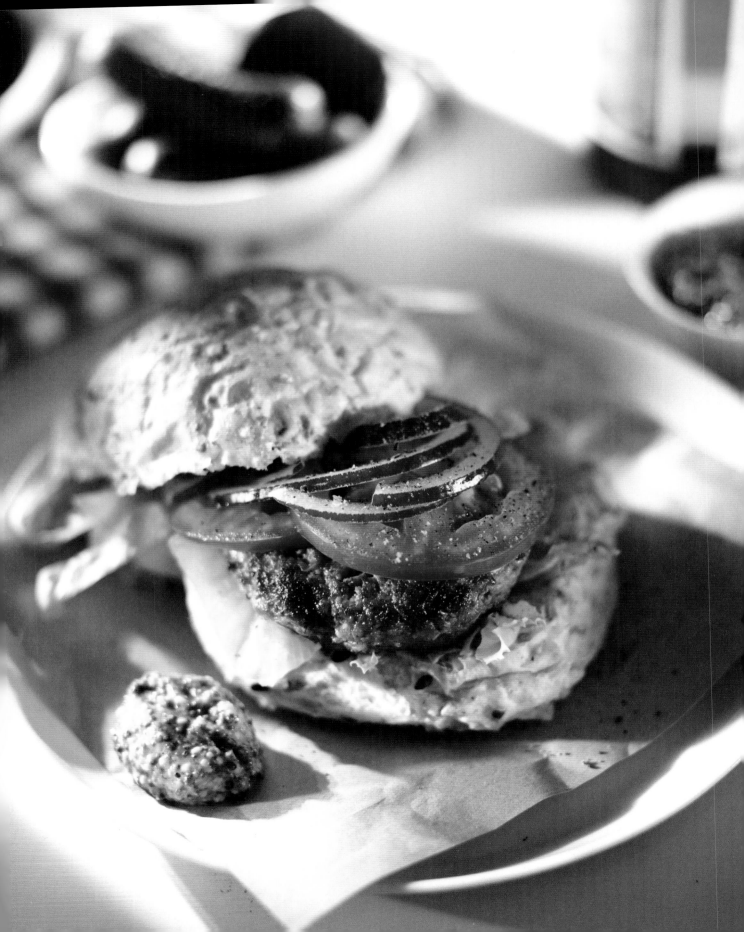

Build your own burger

1 medium carrot, chopped finely

1 medium onion, chopped finely

1 tsp garlic puree

1 stalk celery, trimmed and chopped finely

500g lean beef mince

1 tbsp olive oil

4 grainy rolls or wholemeal hamburger buns

2 cups shredded lettuce

1 large tomato, thinly sliced

1 In a large bowl combine carrot, onion, garlic, celery, mince and 1 teaspoon of the oil. Form into eight patties.
2 Heat the remaining oil in a large frying pan and cook the burgers for 4 minutes on each side, or until cooked through.
3 Serve in a grainy roll or hamburger bun with shredded lettuce, a slice or two of tomato and your favourite condiments.

Yes, burgers really can be a healthy option for a light meal. And they won't break the count budget as long as you keep an eye on the fillings and extras.

Condiment counts

1 TSP MUSTARD: 1

1 TBSP BARBECUE SAUCE: 2

1 TBSP TOMATO SAUCE: 1

1 TBSP 97% FAT-FREE MAYONNAISE: 1

Extra fillings counts

2 SLICES CANNED BEETROOT: 1

4 SLICES PICKLED GHERKINS: 1

2 UNCOOKED ONION RINGS: 0

2 TBSP FRIED ONION RINGS: 1

'With the works'

1 EGG (PAN-FRIED IN MINIMUM OIL): 3

1 SLICE REDUCED-FAT CHEESE: 3

PREP: 10 mins
COOK: 8 mins
SERVES: 4
COUNTS PER SERVE: 19

Tandoori lamb cutlets with tomato and coriander salsa

1 packet butter chicken recipe mix

¾ cup reduced-fat plain yoghurt

12 lamb cutlets, fat trimmed

Tomato and coriander salsa

2 tsp canola oil

1 small red onion, peeled and finely chopped

2 large ripe tomatoes, chopped

1 tbsp lemon or lime juice

1 tbsp sweet chilli sauce

2 tbsp chopped coriander leaves

1 Combine the butter chicken recipe mix with the yoghurt and use it to marinate the lamb cutlets. Place the cutlets in a covered dish in the fridge for 20 minutes, or until you are ready to cook.
2 While the meat is marinating, combine all the salsa ingredients and mix well.
3 Preheat the grill or barbecue. Grill or barbecue the cutlets for 2–3 minutes a side, depending on thickness. Serve with salsa.

We like to serve these cutlets at a weekend barbecue with a scoop of rice and a crispy green salad. If time allows, rest for 5 minutes under a foil covering before serving.

PREP: 10 mins
MARINATE: 20 mins
COOK: 6 mins
SERVES: 6
COUNTS PER SERVE: 15
½ CUP COOKED RICE: 5 counts

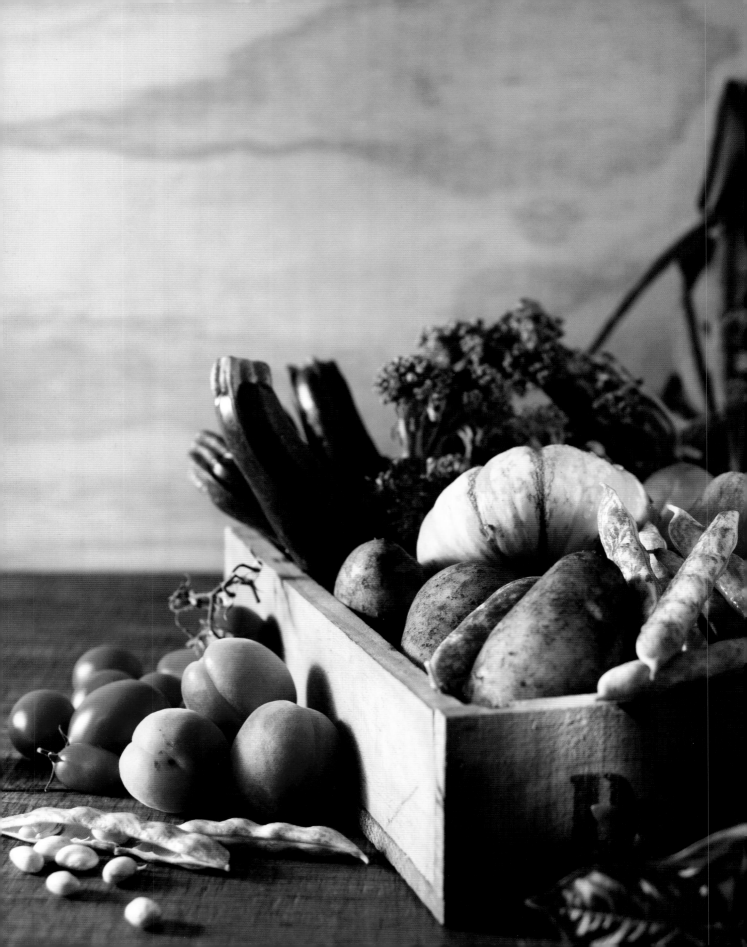

Getting dinner on the table at the end of the day can be a challenge with tired children, work-weary partners and fussy eaters to contend with. But this main meal matters because it's usually the day's biggest meal and an opportunity to eat a wide variety of foods (especially those vital vegetables). It's more than that, too. It's a chance for the family to come together and reconnect.

The food lover's way to a healthy dinner

Reconnect: Chatting about the day's events and coming together as a family or catching up with friends can be the best part of dinner.

Encourage: Sitting down at the table as a family encourages kids to try more vegetables and new foods, and helps build healthy habits (and good table manners) for a lifetime. If you have fussy eaters in your family, they are more likely to try new foods and eat their greens if you involve them in choosing and preparing dinner.

Enjoy: Sharing stories and laughter, and enjoying being together around the table is a great way to build strong family ties and happy memories.

It's good to remember: Take the time to really enjoy this special meal by turning off distractions such as television and telephones. A satisfying dinner will be around 25 to 35 counts.

Q&A

Q: I truly have no time to cook. How, then, do I avoid resorting to unhealthy takeaway food?

A: You're not alone. These days the family cook typically has 30 minutes or less to whip up something healthy and filling that everyone will eat. Here are some tips:

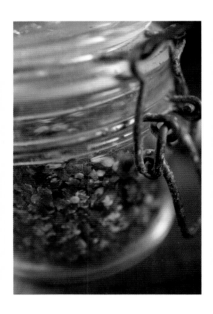

- Keep it quick and simple with healthy foods. You don't have to pull out the recipe book every night. There's nothing wrong with grilled meat, chicken or fish served with a potato or two and plenty of cooked vegetables or a big salad.
- Make the most of 'no time' back-up ingredients—pre-cut vegetables (fresh or frozen), bags of salad, diced meats, slices of cold meats, pre-made sauces and recipe mixes.
- Add some lean mince and chopped onion to a jar of tomato sauce and you have savoury mince, or tacos, or spaghetti bolognaise. Transform the same sauce into chilli con carne with a can of kidney beans, a dash of chilli and some freshly chopped coriander.
- Leave more ambitious recipes for weekends, or those days when you have more time to plan and cook.
- Make the most of your freezer—freeze leftovers and make meals to freeze when you have the time.
- Throw together a big salad while you heat up a frozen pizza with the Heart Foundation Tick for a quick, easy meal that everyone will love. The counts are approx 15 counts per serving—that's an eighth of a regular-size pizza.
- Stock up on frozen meals for those times when you are too tired to do anything but throw something in the microwave (there are plenty of healthy ones like LEAN CUISINE with 12–20 counts per serving).
- Be prepared. Take 30 minutes one day a week to plan at least four or five of the meals for the coming week and write a list for a big supermarket shop. In the long run, this will save both time and money.

Dinner basics—as easy as 1, 2, 3

For most of us, dinner is probably meat (or chicken or fish) with vegetables and potato (or rice or pasta). This is a good place to start when building a healthy meal, but most important is making sure you get the portions right. And this is where the simple 1, 2, 3 plate model can help. Here's how you do it:

1 Eat ONE portion of protein foods like meat, chicken, fish or tofu, which should fit neatly into a quarter of your dinner plate.
2 Eat TWO small portions of starchy carbohydrate foods like potato, sweet potato, pasta, noodles, rice, couscous, cracked wheat, sweetcorn, legumes or bread. As with protein, they should fit into a quarter of your plate.
3 Eat THREE portions of non-starchy vegetables, which should fill up the remaining half of your plate. Think colour and variety with vegetables—we show you how on page 109.

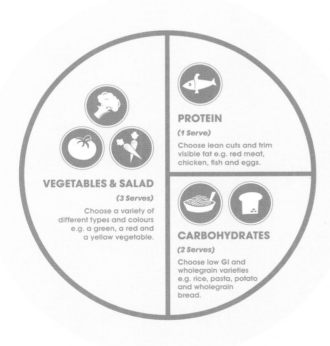

VEGETABLES & SALAD
(3 Serves)
Choose a variety of different types and colours e.g. a green, a red and a yellow vegetable.

PROTEIN
(1 Serve)
Choose lean cuts and trim visible fat e.g. red meat, chicken, fish and eggs.

CARBOHYDRATES
(2 Serves)
Choose low GI and wholegrain varieties e.g. rice, pasta, potato and wholegrain bread.

Protein priorities

Protein foods like meat, chicken, fish, eggs, legumes and nuts are packed with nutrients and are one of the most important building blocks for a healthy body. Protein also helps you to feel fuller for longer, which is great if you want to cut back on snacks.

Priority # 1: Keep it lean

Trimming the fat off meat and choosing the 'skinless' option with chicken cuts the counts and the cholesterol.

Priority # 2: Portion matters

As most of us eat more than enough protein each day to meet our needs, we only need a small amount for dinner. The amount of meat or chicken should be roughly equivalent to the size and thickness of the palm of your hand (no fingers included), and slightly bigger for fish.

Priority # 3: Variety matters, too

Enjoy meat-free meals by substituting with plant protein. Dried beans, split peas and lentils are now all available in more convenient canned, pre-prepared or chilled forms. Tofu and lentil burgers are also widely available. Combine these proteins with nuts, seeds and grains and you can get all the nutrients you need in a vegetarian diet.

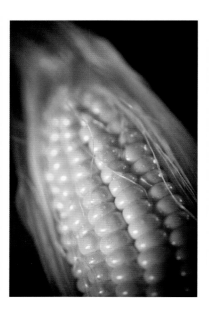

SWEETCORN AND LEGUMES—WHERE DO THEY FIT ON YOUR PLATE?

We've put corn in with the starchy carbohydrates because it's actually a grain and provides energy-giving carbohydrate. But it also includes many of the same important nutrients that vegetables do—so that makes it a great vegetable choice, too!

As for legumes such as peas and beans, they are the perfect all-rounders. We have included them in the protein section to expand your options for meatless meals, but they also contain carbohydrate and provide many of the same important nutrients as vegetables, including being very rich in fibre.

Carbohydrates: the energy givers

Starchy foods like rice, pasta, noodles and bread, or vegetables like potatoes, sweet potatoes and corn, are energy givers. Unless we are athletes, are very active or do heavy physical work, most of us only need a couple of small portions. So what do two portions that will fit on a quarter of your plate look like?

- 1 cup of cooked rice, pasta or noodles.
- 1 cup of corn kernels or a cob of corn.
- three to four chat potatoes or 1 cup of mashed potato.

Vegetables

The half-plate of vegetables should be made up of pile-your-plate-high low 'carb' greens and salad vegetables. You can also add into the mix moderate portions of root vegetables like beetroot, carrots, Jerusalem artichokes, parsnips, swedes and turnips, as well as old favourites like frozen or shelled peas and pumpkin, which have a little more starch but are full of fibre and essential nutrients. These are the vegetables that fill you up without adding many counts. That half-plate can take three of your five daily portions.

Not only are vegetables virtually free foods (depending, of course, on how you cook them and the sauces you serve them with), eating plenty of them is linked to better health and wellbeing. People who maintain a healthy weight eat lots of vegetables, including salads, stir fries and vegetable soups.

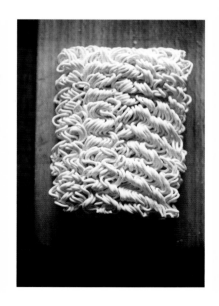

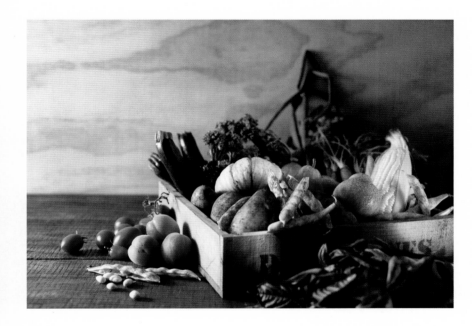

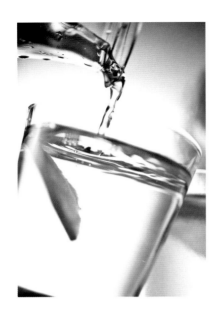

It's OK to cheat

Frozen vegetables are just as good as fresh. We are big fans of frozen peas, beans and corn, and those pre-mixed packs of peas, corn and diced carrot. You can add them to a stir fry, pasta sauce or casserole, or serve them as an accompaniment to lean meat, chicken or fish. Make sure you keep them in your freezer, along with the emergency stir fry vegetable combos.

Dinner for one or two

These mini recipes serve two people, so simply halve the quantities for one or double them for four. The counts given are per individual serving. If you like a sweet finish, a piece of fruit of your choice (apple, pear, large serve of rockmelon) will add 4 counts.

Chicken noodle stir fry

Prepare 125g of fresh thin **egg noodles** according to the packet instructions. Stir fry 250g of sliced skinless **chicken breast fillet** in 2 teaspoons of **oil** for 2–3 minutes. Set aside. Stir fry 1 teaspoon of grated **ginger**, 1 teaspoon of crushed **garlic** and one sliced **onion** for 2 minutes. Add one sliced small **red capsicum** and stir fry for 3 minutes or until just tender. Add three sliced baby **bok choy**, 2 tablespoons of **soy sauce**, ½ teaspoon of **sesame oil** and 1–2 tablespoons of water (if needed). Bring to the boil, add noodles and chicken, and toss to heat through. 15 counts per serve

Meat and three vegetables

Barbecue or char-grill two small, lean **steaks** (around 120g raw weight each) seasoned with a **spice mix** or freshly ground black **pepper**, and serve with (for each person) three baby new **potatoes**, 1 cup of steamed or microwaved **broccoli** florets (or your favourite green vegetable), and one large, ripe **tomato** sliced and drizzled with **balsamic vinegar** and freshly chopped **basil**. 15 counts per serve

Greek salad and tuna

Place in a bowl one medium Lebanese **cucumber** (sliced), two chopped **tomatoes**, half a medium **red onion** (finely sliced), 2 cups of **mesclun mix**, and two or three torn, crisp **cos leaves**. Add six pitted kalamata **olives**, four cubes of **feta**, one hard-boiled **egg** (quartered) and a 185g can of **tuna** in spring water (drained and flaked). Gently toss in 2 tablespoons of **vinaigrette** dressing. If desired, serve with a small (60g) wholegrain dinner roll (add 3 counts). 16 counts per serve

Minestrone with basil pesto

Sauté one sliced **onion** with chopped **garlic** and ¼ cup of diced **bacon** for 5 minutes. Stir in one sliced **celery** stalk, one small diced **carrot**, two chopped **tomatoes** and ½ teaspoon of dried **oregano**. Add 3 cups of vegetable or chicken **stock**, bring to the boil and simmer for 10 minutes. Add ½ cup of **risoni** and ½ cup of canned (drained) **cannellini beans**, and simmer until vegetables and pasta are cooked. Stir in ½ cup of frozen **peas** and 2 teaspoons of basil **pesto**, and heat through. If desired, serve with a piece of wholegrain toast spread with margarine (add 5 counts). 18 counts per serve

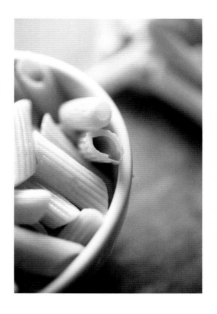

Penne with ricotta and pesto

Cook 150g (about 1½ level cups) **pasta shapes** according to the packet instructions. Mix ½ cup of reduced-fat **ricotta** with 1 tablespoon of **pesto** in a small bowl until smooth (add a little of the pasta cooking water if necessary). Drain the pasta and return to the pan. Stir in 1 tablespoon of **balsamic vinegar**. Mix in the ricotta sauce. Serve topped with 2 tablespoons of grated **parmesan** and a big mixed **garden salad** (2 cups each) tossed in 2 tablespoons of **vinaigrette** dressing. 24 counts per serve

Mix and match your dinner

For a healthy dinner, choose foods from each of the following groups:

- Breads, grains and starchy vegetables.
- Meat, chicken, fish, eggs, dairy foods, nuts, seeds and legumes.
- Vegetables.

For most of us, a satisfying dinner will have around 25 counts. The counts we give here are only average counts for these typical foods. Check out the counts for your favourite foods and brands in our ready-reckoner on page 222.

Typical counts for rice, pasta, noodles
and starchy vegetables like potato

- **2 counts** = ½ cup of mashed pumpkin or a small wedge of baked pumpkin; ¼ cup of croutons.
- **3 counts** = one small cob corn; one thin slice of toast; one small (30g) dinner roll.
- **4 counts** = ¼ cup of breadcrumbs.
- **5 counts** = ½ cup of cooked brown rice.
- **6 counts** = one small tortilla; one medium boiled or steamed potato; four medium baked potato wedges; two pieces of baked sweet potato (200g); one quarter of a regular size pizza base.
- **7 counts** = ⅔ cup of mashed potato with milk; ½ cup of cooked polenta.
- **8 counts** = one large pita pocket bread; 1 cup of cooked couscous; ½ cup of (uncooked) gnocci.
- **9 counts** = ½ cup of potato salad; 1 cup of cooked rice; 1 cup of cooked noodles; half a round naan bread.
- **10 counts** = 1 cup of cooked pasta.

Typical counts for meat, chicken, fish, dairy foods,
eggs and legumes

Note: Fresh meat, chicken and fish are grilled unless otherwise stated. Add 2 counts extra for each teaspoon of oil used for pan-frying.

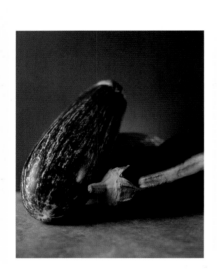

- **3 counts** = one small can of tuna in spring water (drained); one grilled fish finger; twelve large cooked and shelled prawns.
- **4 counts** = one large (53g) egg (boiled or poached); one thin low-fat (8%) grilled sausage; three slices of smoked salmon; one dozen fresh oysters.
- **5 counts** = one small (130g) can of baked beans or one small (125g) can of chickpeas or lentils (drained); two large, thick slices of ham off the bone, trimmed; one thin reduced-fat (15%) grilled sausage; one medium lamb cutlet (uncooked); two small slices of roast lean beef; one grilled fish fillet; one crab/seafood stick; 100g firm (plain) tofu.
- **6 counts** = ⅓ cup of grated light cheese; one thin grilled sausage; one grilled or barbecued satay chicken kebab.
- **7 counts** = half a grilled skinless chicken breast fillet; one grilled rissole or hamburger pattie made with lean mince.

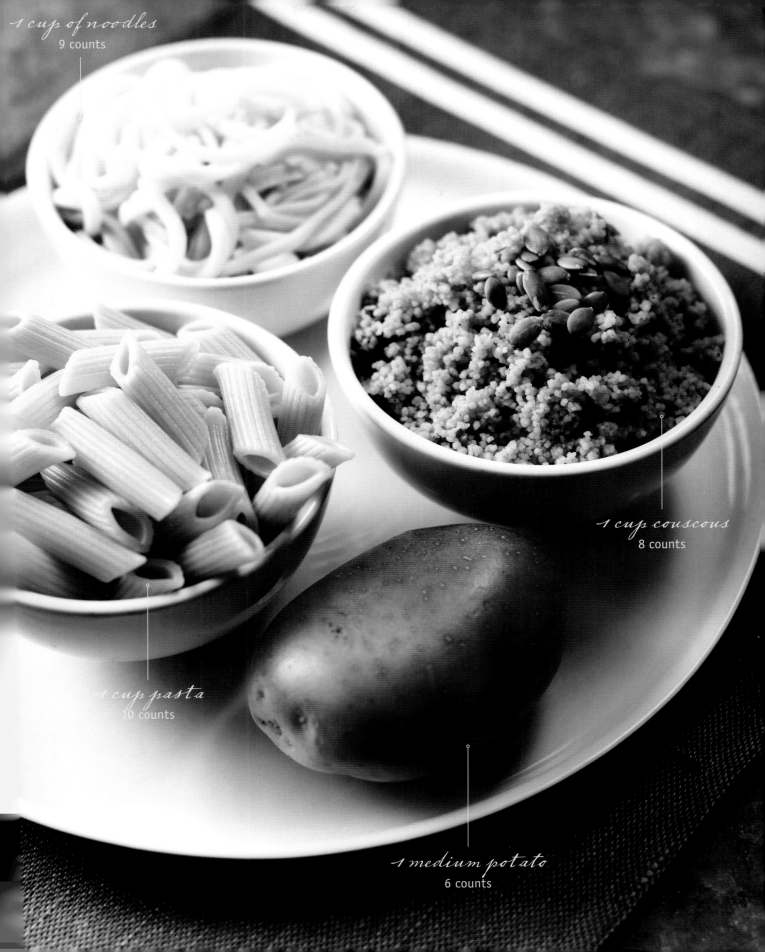

1 cup of noodles
9 counts

1 cup couscous
8 counts

1 cup pasta
10 counts

1 medium potato
6 counts

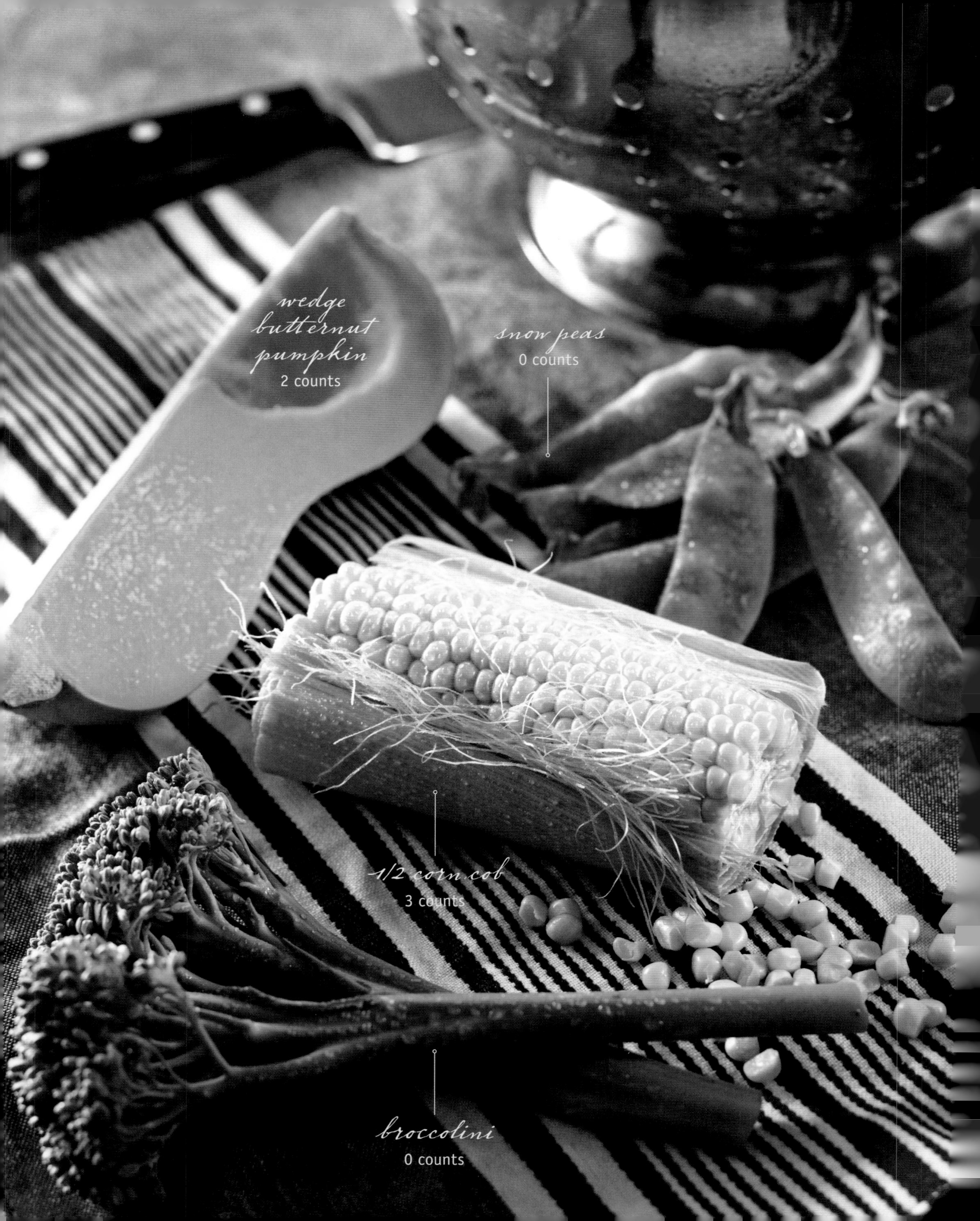

wedge
butternut
pumpkin
2 counts

snow peas
0 counts

1/2 corn cob
3 counts

broccolini
0 counts

- **8 counts** = one small crumbed and oven-baked fish fillet; one small grilled mid-loin pork chop, fat trimmed; two lean slices of roast lamb; 100g marinated tofu.
- **9 counts** = one small piece (100g) of lean grilled steak; one medium (100g) grilled skinless chicken thigh fillet.
- **13 counts** = two well-trimmed, grilled lamb loin chops; one large baked chicken drumstick (with skin); one small lean schnitzel, crumbed and lightly pan-fried.
- **14 counts** = one quarter of a small quiche, one small piece of barbecued chicken drumstick and thigh (with skin).
- **17 counts** = two small, thick (22% fat) grilled sausages.
- **19 counts** = one large slice of homemade quiche with pastry base.

Typical counts for vegetables

Colour your plate with bonus vegetables. All these vegetables have less than 1 count in the quantities most people eat them, so have plenty on your plate and enjoy them for free. (If juicing or blending for soup, some vegetables, like pumpkin, peas and carrot, will need to be included in the counts as they are a source of carbohydrate. They will also need to be added to the total counts in recipes where they are used as a main ingredient, not just an accompaniment.)

Green: artichokes, Asian greens, asparagus, avocados, green beans, bok choy, broccoli, broccolini, brussels sprouts, cabbage, Chinese cabbage, green capsicum, celery, chard, chicory, choko, choy sum, cress, cucumber, endive, leafy greens, leeks, lettuce, mesclun, okra, peas (including snow peas and sugar snap peas), rocket, silverbeet, spinach, spring onions, squash, watercress, witlof, zucchini.

Red/pink: red capsicum, radishes, Spanish onions, tomatoes.

White/cream: bamboo shoots, cauliflower, celeriac, daikon, fennel, garlic, Jerusalem artichoke, kohlrabi, mushrooms, onions, parsnips, shallots, swedes, turnips, white corn.

Orange/yellow: butternut squash, yellow/orange capsicum, carrots, pumpkin, squash, winter squash, yellow beets, yellow tomatoes.

Blue/purple: beetroot, eggplant, purple asparagus, radicchio lettuce, red cabbage.

See page 79 for salad vegetables.

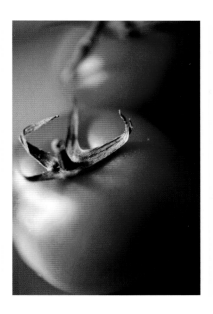

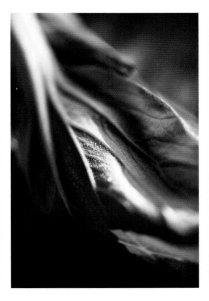

It's good to remember: Our preference is to steam our bonus vegetables. Add 2 counts per teaspoon if pan-frying in oil.

Typical counts for fats and oils

Note: Teaspoon and tablespoon measures are level. Heap it and you are adding extra counts.

- **2 counts** = 1 teaspoon of cooking oil, butter or margarine; 1 tablespoon of hummus; 1 tablespoon of pesto; 1 tablespoon of satay peanut sauce.
- **3 counts** = 1 tablespoon of vinaigrette; 1 tablespoon of sundried tomatoes in vegetable oil (drained).
- **4 counts** = 1 tablespoon of spicy green tapenade.
- **5 counts** = 1 tablespoon of hollandaise sauce; 1 tablespoon of taramasalata; half a small avacado.
- **7 counts** = 1 tablespoon of regular mayonnaise; 1 tablespoon of garlic butter.

Typical counts for condiments

- **Free** = ground pepper; fresh and dried herbs; curry powder; 1 teaspoon of soy sauce; mustard; balsamic vinegar; lemon juice; fat-free salad dressings; 1 teaspoon of horseradish cream; 1 teaspoon of cranberry sauce.
- **1 count** = 1 tablespoon of Worcestershire sauce; ½ tablespoon of tomato or barbecue sauce; 1 tablespoon of curry paste; 3 tablespoons of gravy; 1 tablespoon of béarnaise sauce.
- **2 counts** = 1 tablespoon of fruit chutney or pickle or relish; 1 tablespoon of sweet chilli sauce; 1 tablespoon of cheese sauce, 1 tablespoon of cranberry sauce.
- **3 counts** = 1 tablespoon of mint jelly.

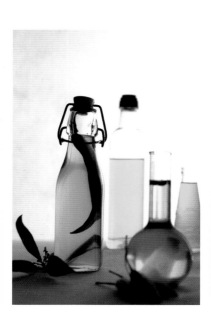

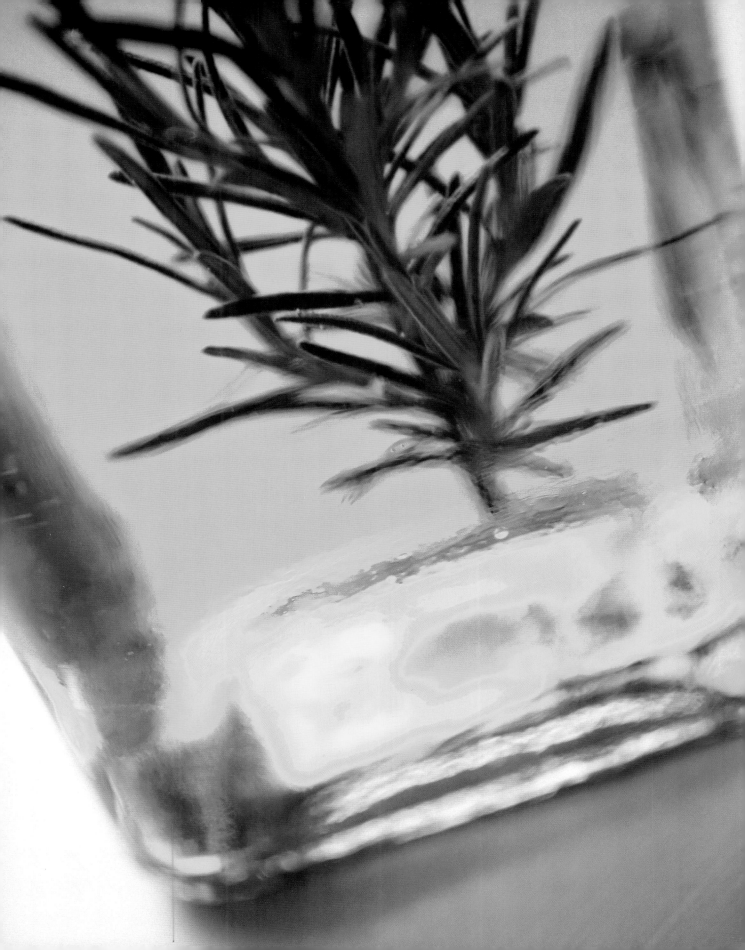

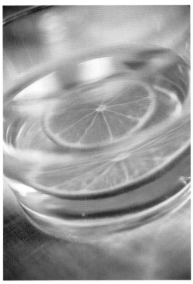

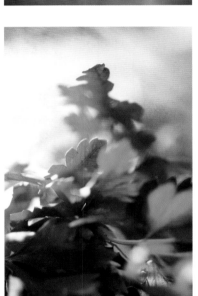

COOKING COUNTS

The way in which you prepare your meal does matter. Different cooking methods can add extra counts that mean you have to cut back in other areas.

If you eat 150g chat (baby new) potatoes:

- Boiled or steamed = 6 counts.
- Mashed with margarine and milk = 8 counts.
- Fried as chips = 22 counts.

If you eat 1 cup cooked pasta:

- Boiled until al dente =10 counts.
- Plus ¾ cup ready-made tomato pasta sauce = 17 counts.
- Plus ¾ cup ready-made bolognaise sauce = 19 counts.
- Plus ¾ cup ready-made cheesy Alfredo sauce = 29 counts.

If you eat 100g chicken thigh fillet:

- Skinless, roasted = 9 counts.
- Skin on, roasted = 11 counts.
- Skinless, crumbed and fried = 18 counts.

Eating out

If you dine out occasionally or only on special occasions, then just enjoy yourself. If you eat out regularly, you need to make sure your choices don't cause a blow-out in your diet. Here are some hints and tips to help guide your choices:

- Make sure you drink plenty of tap water as it can help make you feel full—other drinks like soft drinks, juices and alcohol will add more counts to your meal.
- The meal extras like bread with butter or oil will add extra counts, so only eat them if you are really hungry and you have the spare counts.
- Stir fries are a better choice than creamy curries.
- Grilled or char-grilled food generally has less counts than deep-fried or pan-fried food.
- A tomato-based pasta would be a better choice than a creamy sauce.
- If you aren't very hungry, consider ordering an entrée size for your main meal.

- The best side to order would be a leafy salad or vegetables as they won't add too many counts to your meal.
- Vegetables, salad or boiled potatoes are better choices then fried chips.
- You don't need to finish everything on your plate—you can always take part of the meal home for lunch the next day.
- Share a dessert or choose fresh fruit or fruit sorbet at the end of the meal.
- Eat your meal slowly and talk to those around you as it will help you eat less.
- Enjoy a walk after dinner.

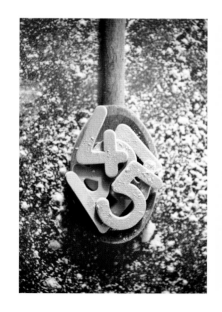

Count the difference with the meal deals

Look how the cost of convenience can add to your daily counts total. To save counts:

CHOOSE THIS	INSTEAD OF THIS
LEAN CUISINE (Honey Soy Beef With Wholemeal Noodles) = 12 counts	McCain (Red Box) Chicken Fettuccine = 28 counts
Hungry Jack's Grilled Chicken Burger = 16 counts	Hungry Jack's Double Whopper with cheese = 49 counts
Subway (9cm) roasted beef with ranch dressing and cheese = 18 counts	Subway (15cm) Meatball Marinara with ranch dressing = 26 counts
Half a frozen Papa Giuseppi's Tropical Supremo Pizza with National Heart Foundation Tick = 27 counts	Half a takeaway pizza 'BBQ meat lovers' = 48 counts
Nando's Classic Chicken Wrap = 13 counts	Nando's Supremo steak = 27 With chips = 51
Sumo Salad Grilled Chicken Caesar Salad = 19 counts	Sumo Salad Chicken Caesar Wrap = 31 counts
3 homemade filled tacos made according to packet instructions = 26 counts	Café-style nachos with cheese, beans, tomato salsa and sour cream = 44 counts
Takeaway grilled fish (150g) = 7 counts	Takeaway battered fish (150g) = 18 counts
1 cup boiled white rice = 9 counts	1 cup fried rice = 17 counts

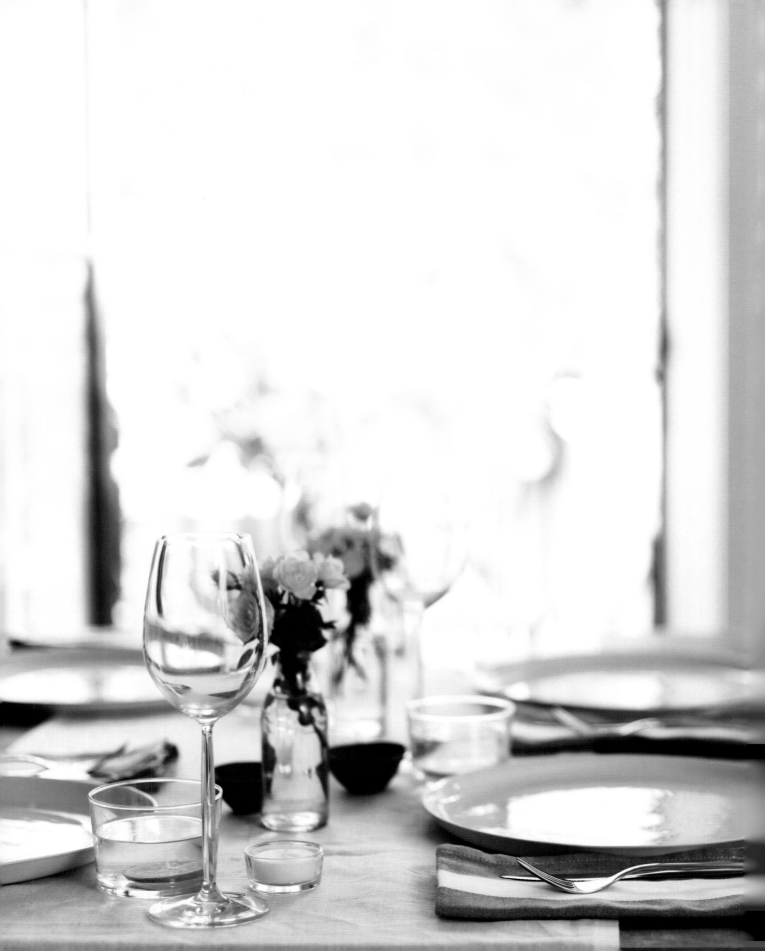

Healthy dinner recipes

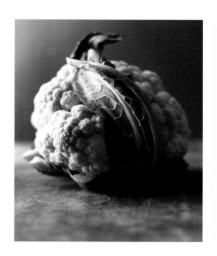

Easy bolognaise sauce

1 tsp olive oil

500g lean beef mince

1 medium carrot, finely diced

1 cup mushrooms, finely diced

1 stalk celery, finely diced

1 medium red capsicum, finely diced

1 medium onion, finely diced

1 tsp fresh rosemary, chopped

1 tsp picked thyme leaves

2 cloves garlic, crushed

400g can chopped tomatoes

⅓ cup tomato paste

½ cup beef stock

1 tsp brown sugar

1 Heat the oil in a large frying pan, add the mince and cook, stirring with a wooden spoon to break up the mince, for 5 minutes or until browned. Add the carrot, mushrooms, celery, capsicum, onion, rosemary, thyme and garlic, and cook for another 5 minutes.

2 Add the tomatoes, tomato paste, beef stock and sugar to the pan. Bring to the boil, then reduce the heat, cover and cook for another 15 minutes.

We have made this with fresh herbs but, of course, you can substitute with dried—just use a little less (½ teaspoon). You may be surprised to see sugar in a savoury recipe, but it really brings out the flavour of the tomatoes. Serve with spaghetti or your favourite pasta shapes, and a crispy green salad or a tomato and basil salad.

PREP: 20 mins
COOK: 25 mins
SERVES: 6
COUNTS PER SERVE: 8
1 CUP COOKED PASTA: 10 counts

With this versatile meat mix we show you how to make meatballs and patties (burgers), and sneak extra vegetables (chop them very, very finely or grate them if you prefer) onto the dinner plate without anyone noticing. In fact, don't be surprised if they come back for seconds. You could also use this mix to make meatloaf.

PREP: 15 mins
REST: 30 mins (meatballs)
COOK: 6–8 mins
MAKES: about 16 meatballs
or 8 patties
COUNTS (1 PATTIE): 6
COUNTS (1 MEATBALL): 3

You need something to mop up the delicious sauce from this quick and easy stroganoff, so serve with mashed potato or sweet potato, rice or pasta, plus plenty of green vegetables or a crispy garden salad.

PREP: 15 mins
COOK: 15 mins
SERVES: 4
COUNTS PER SERVE: 14
½ CUP COOKED RICE: 5 counts
½ CUP MASHED POTATO: 4 counts

Magic mince for meatballs or patties

1 medium carrot, peeled and finely chopped or grated

1 medium onion, finely chopped

1 tsp garlic puree

1 stalk celery, trimmed and sliced finely

500g lean beef mince

1 tsp olive oil

1 In a large bowl combine the carrot, onion, garlic, celery, mince and oil, and follow one of the methods below.

2 To make meatballs, roll level tablespoons of the mixture into balls, place on a plate or tray and chill, covered, for 30 minutes in the refrigerator. To pan-fry, heat 1 teaspoon of oil in a large frying pan and cook the meatballs for 3 minutes on each side, or until cooked through. To simmer the meatballs in a quick tomato sauce, add 3 tablespoons of tomato paste to one can (400g) of chopped tomatoes and simmer the meatballs until cooked (about 15–20 minutes).

3 To make burgers, form the mix into eight small patties, each about 6–7cm in diameter. Heat some oil in a large frying pan and cook the burgers for 4 minutes on each side, or until done. Serve in a roll with your favourite burger toppings.

Quick and easy beef stroganoff

2 tsp olive oil

500g tender beef strips

1 clove garlic, crushed

1 small onion, chopped

100g mushrooms, sliced

1 tbsp tomato paste

3 tsp beef stock powder

375ml CARNATION Light & Creamy Evaporated Milk

1 tbsp cornflour

1 Heat the oil in a large non-stick frying pan and brown the beef strips. Remove from the pan and set aside, keeping warm. Add the garlic, onion and mushrooms to the pan, and cook, stirring, for 2 minutes.

2 Mix together the tomato paste, stock powder, evaporated milk and cornflour, add to the pan and bring to the boil, stirring. Add the beef strips, then reduce the heat and simmer for 5 minutes or until heated through, stirring occasionally.

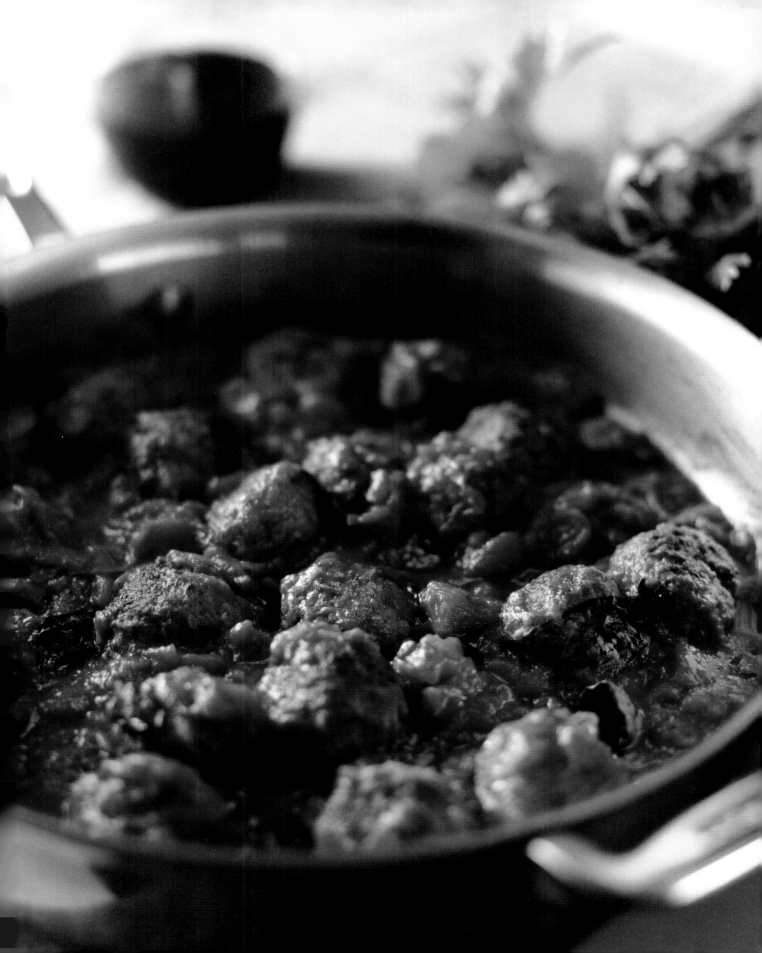

Spicy beef and noodle salad

PREP: 20 mins
COOK: 10 mins
REST: 5 mins
SERVES: 4
COUNTS PER SERVE: 19

olive or canola oil spray

300g rump steak

2 tbsp sweet chilli sauce

⅔ cup low-fat French dressing

1 tbsp chopped fresh basil or mint leaves

700g fresh Hokkien noodles

1 green capsicum, thinly sliced

1 red capsicum, thinly sliced

150g snow peas, halved

250g punnet cherry tomatoes, halved

1 Lebanese cucumber, thinly sliced into rounds

1 Spray a wok or non-stick frying pan with oil, and heat. Cook the steak over medium heat for 3 minutes on each side. Remove from the wok, wrap in foil and set aside for 5 minutes before slicing thinly. Place in a serving bowl.
2 Combine the sweet chilli sauce with the dressing and basil in a small bowl.
3 Prepare the noodles according to the packet instructions, then separate with two forks. Drain thoroughly.
4 While the noodles are still warm, combine with the steak, dressing and vegetables. Toss thoroughly, then serve immediately.

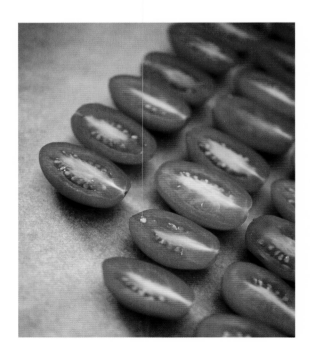

Lamb biryani

olive or canola oil spray

1 medium onion, chopped

2 tsp minced garlic

1 tbsp minced ginger

2 tbsp Indian curry paste

1 tsp cumin, ground

1 tsp cinnamon, ground

1 tsp turmeric, ground

2 tsp coriander, ground

500g lean lamb, cubed

1½ cups basmati rice

4 cups chicken stock

1 cup frozen peas

2 cups cauliflower florets

¼ cup chopped dried apricots

To serve

200g tub low-fat plain yoghurt

2 tbsp chopped fresh mint

2 tomatoes, chopped

2 tbsp chopped fresh coriander

*A biryani is like a pilaf—
a dish of meat, rice,
vegetables and aromatic
spices. It's an ideal one-
dish dinner served with
side dishes like yoghurt
and mint, and tomatoes
and coriander. Use your
favourite curry paste to
make the biryani—Madras
or tikka work well.*

PREP: 15 mins
COOK: 40 mins
REST: 5 mins
SERVES: 6
COUNTS PER SERVE: 18

1 Preheat the oven to 180°C (160°C fan-forced). Spray a large ovenproof casserole dish with oil and cook the onion and garlic over medium heat until soft. Add the ginger, curry paste, cumin, cinnamon, turmeric and ground coriander, and cook, stirring, for 1 minute. Add ⅓ cup water, if necessary, to prevent sticking. Add lamb and cook for 3–5 minutes, or until browned.

2 Stir in the rice and cook for 1 minute. Add stock, peas, cauliflower and apricots, and bring to a simmer.

3 Cover the dish and bake in the oven for 25–30 minutes, or until the stock is absorbed and the rice is cooked. Remove from the oven and allow to rest for 5 minutes before serving.

4 Combine the yoghurt and mint in one small bowl, and in another bowl combine the tomatoes and coriander. Serve the biryani with the yoghurt mixture and tomato mixture on the side.

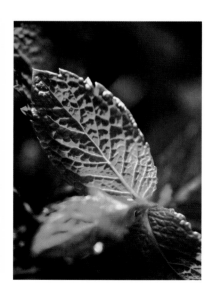

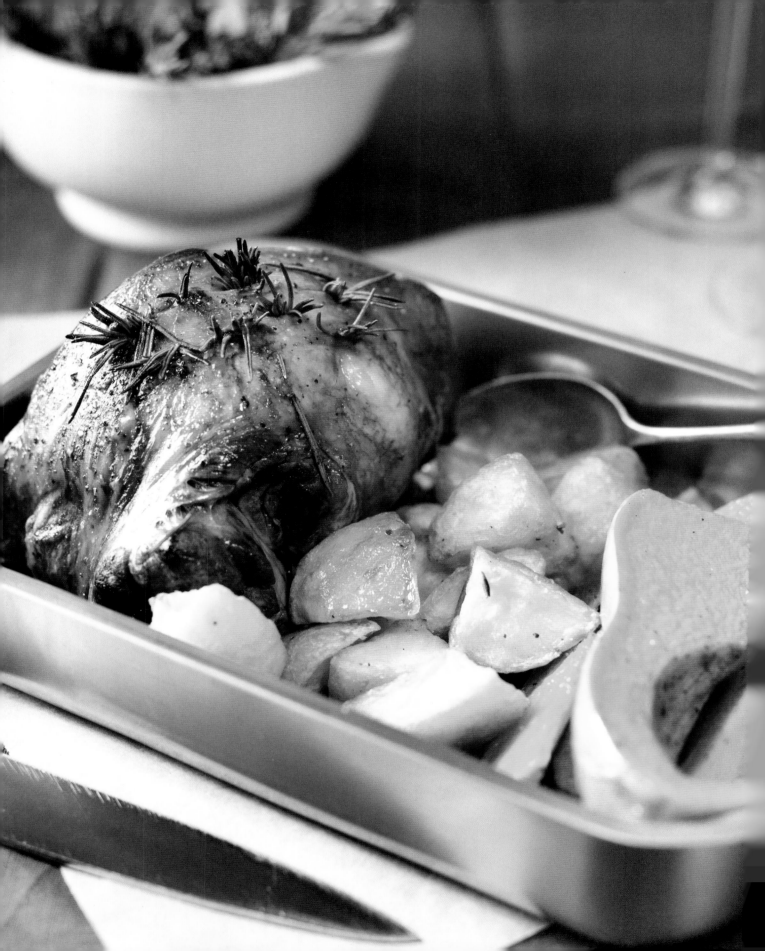

Easy-carve roast lamb with vegetables and onion gravy

880g easy-carve mini lamb roast

500g pumpkin, peeled and cut into chunks

6 small potatoes (120g each), peeled and halved

2 tbsp oil

1 packet MAGGI Brown Onion Gravy Mix

¼ cup red wine

¼ tsp rosemary leaves, chopped

1 Preheat the oven to 220°C (200°C fan-forced).
2 Lightly brush the lamb and vegetable pieces with oil, and place in a baking dish. Bake in the oven for 20 minutes, then reduce the temperature to 190°C (170°C fan-forced). Cook for a further 45 minutes, turning the vegetables three times during cooking. Remove from the oven, cover loosely with foil and rest for 5–10 minutes before carving.
3 Make up the gravy mix according to the packet instructions, with 1 cup of water and the wine and rosemary.
4 Serve the sliced lamb with roasted vegetables, gravy and plenty of green vegetables.

Easy-carve lamb roast is a simple meal because it looks after itself in the oven. And because it is already boned, carving it is easy too. Set it aside, covered with foil, to stand for 10 minutes before carving. Serve with your favourite streamed green vegetables and don't forget the mint sauce or mint jelly.

PREP: 15 mins
COOK: 65 mins
REST: 10 mins
SERVES: 6
COUNTS PER SERVE: 23

Chilli pork stir fry

canola oil spray

200g lean pork mince

1 packet MAGGI 99% fat free 2 Minute Noodles, Chicken Flavour

2 cups snow peas, sliced lengthways

4 cups bean sprouts

2 tbsp sweet chilli sauce

1 tbsp fish sauce

1 Spray a non-stick frying pan with oil and stir fry the pork for 2 minutes.
2 Prepare the noodles according to the packet instructions. When the noodles have 1 minute to go, add the snow peas and bean sprouts to the pork, and stir fry for 1 minute.
3 Remove from the heat, stir through the drained noodles, and sweet chilli and fish sauces, and serve.

This simple stir fry is not only a complete meal, it really is on the table in just 10 minutes.

PREP: 5 mins
COOK: 5 mins
SERVES: 2
COUNTS PER SERVE: 20

PREP: 10 mins
COOK: 5 mins
SERVES: 4
COUNTS PER SERVE: 12

San choy bau

1 tbsp sesame oil

400g lean pork mince

1 tsp finely chopped ginger

1 clove garlic, crushed

225g can water chestnuts, drained and chopped

225g can bamboo shoots, drained and chopped

1 tbsp fish sauce

2 tbsp oyster sauce

1 tbsp sweet chilli sauce

2 shallots (spring onions), sliced

1 lettuce, outer leaves cut into cups

2 tbsp chopped fresh coriander leaves, to serve

1 Heat the oil in a heavy-based frying pan or a wok, and brown the pork with the ginger and garlic. Add the water chestnuts and bamboo shoots, and stir fry for 1 minute to heat through. Add the fish sauce, oyster sauce, sweet chilli sauce and shallots, and stir through.
2 Spoon the mixture into lettuce cups to serve, sprinkled with coriander.

This is a pretty and vibrant barbecue dish. You need 12 wooden skewers. Pre-soaking the skewers in water for an hour beforehand helps to prevent them from burning on the barbecue.

PREP: 10 mins
CHILL: 20 mins
COOK: 15 mins
MAKES: 12 skewers
COUNTS PER SKEWER: 3

Chicken and vegetable skewers

400g skinless chicken breast fillet, cut into 2cm cubes

1 packet chicken and mushroom soup mix

12 large button mushrooms, quartered

24 cherry tomatoes

2 medium zucchini, sliced

1 Toss the chicken in the soup mix, cover and chill for 20 minutes.
2 Preheat the barbecue or grill.
3 Thread the chicken pieces onto the skewers, alternating with the mushrooms, tomatoes and zucchini.
4 Barbecue or grill on a medium heat for 10–15 minutes, turning frequently until cooked.

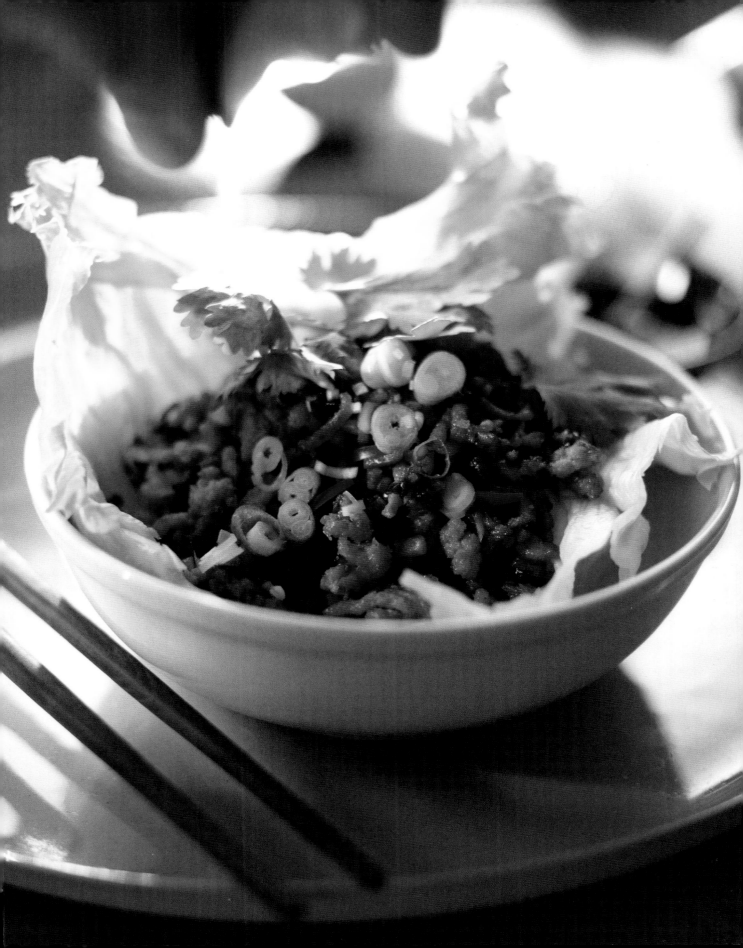

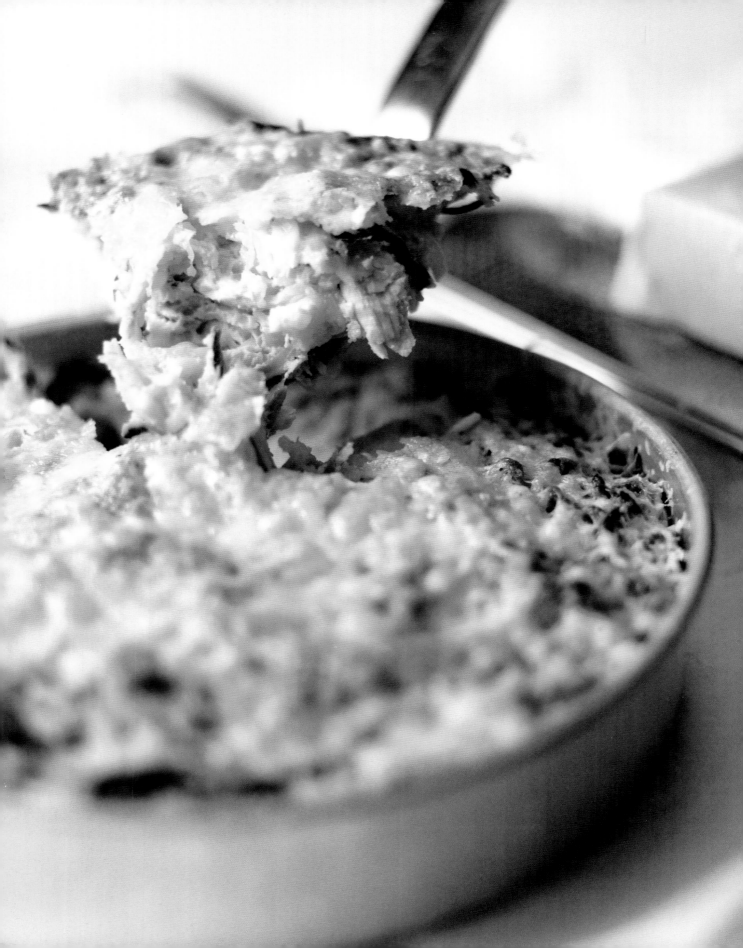

Chicken and corn bake

1 packet MAGGI 2 Minute Noodles, Chicken Flavour

¼ cooked chicken, skin and bones removed, shredded

125g can corn kernels, rinsed and drained

1 zucchini, grated

3 eggs, lightly beaten

½ cup tasty cheese

1 Preheat the oven to 180°C (160°C fan-forced). Grease and line the base of a 20cm round cake tin or ovenproof frying pan.

2 In a saucepan, break the noodle cake into quarters and cover with boiling water. Bring to the boil, simmer for 2 minutes, then drain.

3 Combine the noodles, chicken, corn, zucchini, eggs and contents of the flavour sachet in a bowl. Spoon the mixture into the prepared pan and sprinkle with cheese.

4 Bake for 25 minutes. Turn out of the pan and serve cheese-side up.

This recipe is perfect for using up leftover roasted or takeaway chicken. It's an easy meal, and all you need with it is a mixed-leaf salad tossed in a light vinaigrette dressing. If there are leftovers, it's ideal for your lunch box the next day.

PREP: 10 mins
COOK: 25 mins
SERVES: 4
COUNTS PER SERVE: 14

Apricot chicken

1 tsp olive oil

1 medium onion, sliced

500g skinless chicken breast fillet, diced

1 cup chicken stock

405ml can apricot nectar

½ cup dried apricots, chopped

1 tbsp cornflour, blended with a little water

1 Heat the oil in a medium frying pan and cook the onion for 2 minutes, or until golden. Add the chicken and cook for a further 2 minutes. Add the stock, apricot nectar and dried apricots, and cook for 5 minutes. Finally, add blended cornflour and water to the pan and stir until the mixture boils and thickens slightly.

This quick and easy apricot chicken dish is on the table in 20 minutes. Serve with rice and your favourite green vegetables, or a salad.

PREP: 10 mins
COOK: 10 mins
SERVES: 4
COUNTS PER SERVE: 14
½ CUP COOKED RICE: 5 counts

You can make this as a
single large pie rather
than individual pies if
you prefer. Serve it with a
crispy garden salad.

PREP: 10 mins
COOK: 30 mins
SERVES: 4
COUNTS PER SERVE: 20

Chicken and filo pies

olive or canola oil spray

500g skinless chicken breast fillet, cubed

1 leek, sliced

250g mushrooms, quartered

1 medium red capsicum, chopped

1 packet chicken and mushroom soup mix

375ml CARNATION Light & Creamy Evaporated Milk

¼ cup chopped fresh parsley

4 sheets filo pastry

1 tsp sesame seeds

1 Preheat the oven to 180°C (160°C fan-forced).

2 Spray a large, non-stick frying pan with oil and heat. Add the chicken
and lightly brown before adding the leek, mushrooms and capsicum.
Cook for a further 2 minutes, stirring.

3 Combine the soup mix and evaporated milk, and add to the pan.
Bring to the boil, stirring. Add the parsley. Spoon the chicken mixture
into four individual 1-cup ovenproof pie dishes.

4 Lightly spray the filo sheets with oil, scrunch over the top of each
dish and sprinkle the sesame seeds on top. Bake the pies in the oven
for 20 minutes, or until the pastry is golden.

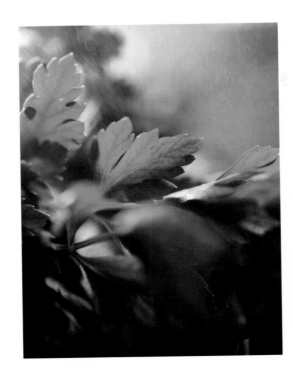

THE FOOD LOVER'S DIET

Mexican tortilla soup

olive or canola oil spray

1 onion, diced

1 tsp garlic, minced

1 tsp chilli, minced

500g chicken breast fillet, chopped

1 tsp chilli powder, or to taste

2 tsp ground cumin

1 tsp dried oregano

4 cups chicken stock

400g can tomatoes, coarsely chopped

4 flour tortillas (19cm)

2 tbsp fresh coriander, finely chopped

400g can corn kernels, rinsed and drained

¼ cup grated low-fat cheese

1 Spray a non-stick saucepan with oil and cook the onion, garlic and chilli over medium heat until soft. Add the chicken and cook until browned all over. Add the chilli powder, cumin and oregano, and cook for 1 minute. Add the stock and tomatoes, then reduce heat to low and simmer for 10 minutes, or until chicken is tender.
2 Meanwhile, preheat the grill to medium-high heat and toast the tortillas until crisp. Break into pieces.
3 Add the coriander to the soup and simmer for 5 minutes. Stir the corn kernels through the soup and heat through.
4 Ladle the soup into six bowls and top with the tortilla pieces, cheese and extra coriander.

This spicy tortilla soup is a warm and hearty meal in a bowl that's just as good the next day if there are any leftovers.

PREP: 10 mins
COOK: 20 mins
SERVES: 6
COUNTS PER SERVE: 17

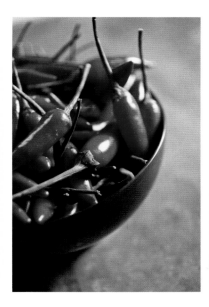

We make this dish with chicken breast fillets, but thigh fillets (all visible fat trimmed) would work just as well and could be more economical.

PREP: 15 mins
COOK: 25 mins
SERVES: 6
COUNTS PER SERVE: 11 (add 2 counts extra for skinless thigh fillets)
½ CUP COOKED RICE = 5 counts

Thai chicken curry

1 tsp peanut or canola oil

500g chicken breast fillets, sliced

1 medium onion, cut into thin wedges

2 slender (finger) eggplants, thinly sliced

2 tbsp red curry paste

375ml light coconut milk

1 tsp chicken stock powder

100g green beans, trimmed and cut in half

1 red capsicum, thinly sliced

1 tbsp fish sauce

juice of half a lime

2 tsp brown sugar

2 tbsp fresh coriander leaves

1 Heat the oil in a wok or large frying pan. Add the chicken, onion and eggplant, and cook over medium heat for 5 minutes. Add the curry paste and cook for 1 minute. Stir in the coconut milk and stock powder, and bring to the boil. Add the beans and capsicum, and simmer, uncovered, for 15 minutes, or until the chicken has cooked through, stirring occasionally.
2 Add the fish sauce, lime juice and sugar to the curry.
3 Serve sprinkled with coriander.

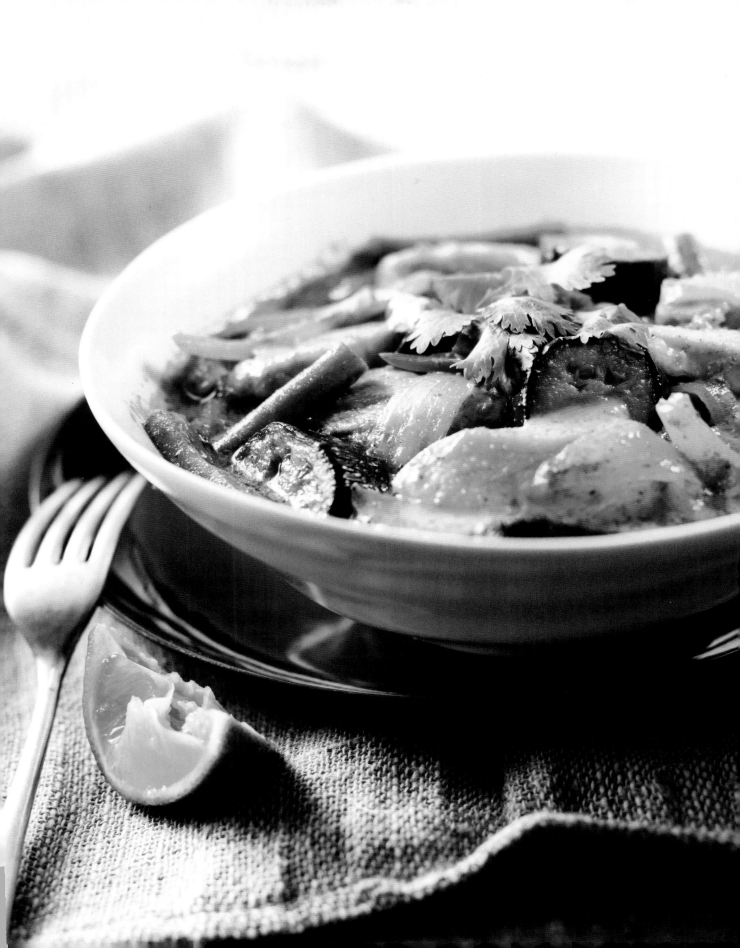

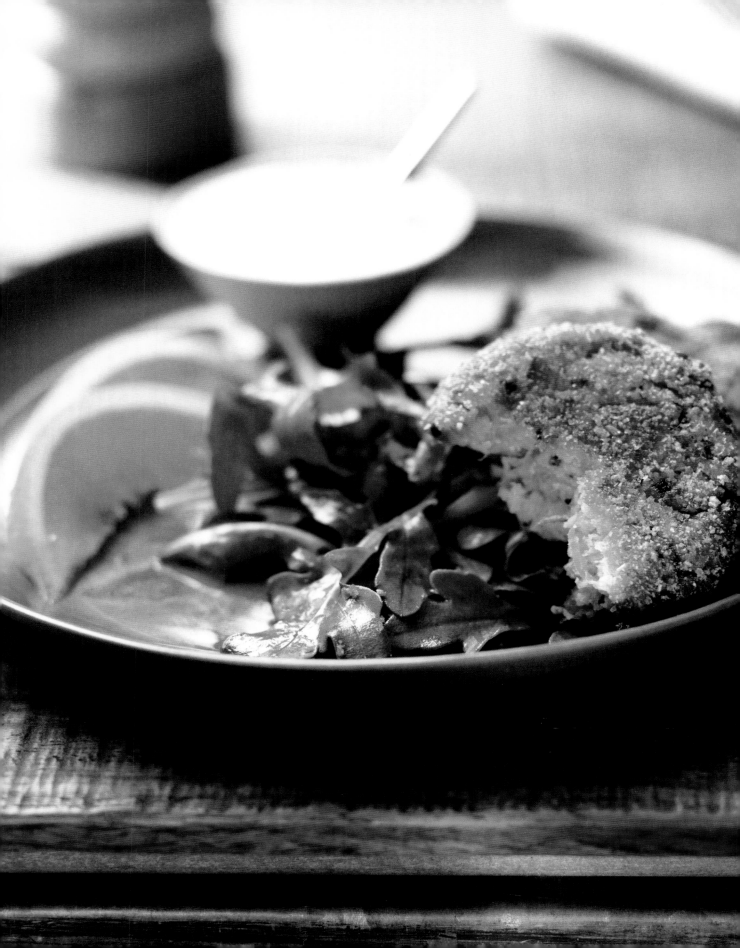

Salmon patties with minty yoghurt sauce

210g can red or pink salmon, drained and bones removed

1 small carrot, grated

1 small zucchini, grated

1 medium tomato, finely chopped

1 tbsp lemon juice

¼ cup powdered milk

½ cup instant potato flakes

1 tbsp dry breadcrumbs

1 tsp seeded mustard

1 egg, lightly beaten

ground black pepper

dry breadcrumbs, extra

Minty yoghurt sauce

⅓ cup light sour cream

1 tbsp low-fat natural yoghurt

2 tsp chopped mint

1 Preheat the oven to 200°C (180°C fan-forced). Lightly grease a baking tray.
2 To make the patties, combine all the ingredients except for the extra breadcrumbs and mix well. Divide the mixture evenly into eight portions. Shape into patties and coat with the extra breadcrumbs.
3 Place the patties on the tray and bake for 15 minutes. Turn the patties over and bake for a further 15 minutes.
4 While the patties are cooking, combine all the sauce ingredients. Serve with the salmon patties.

Salmon patties (just like mince patties) are a great way to sneak in extra vegetables. Just make sure you grate them finely. This meal is a pantry special. As an alternative to instant potato flakes, take one large potato and quarter, then steam or microwave and dry mash. Serve with a salad or your favourite green vegetables.

PREP: 20 mins
COOK: 30 mins
SERVES: 4
COUNTS PER SERVE: 12

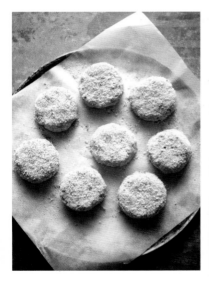

PREP: 15 mins
COOK: 15 mins
SERVES: 8
COUNTS PER SERVE: 15

Seafood and basil stir fry

2 cups long-grain rice

canola or olive oil spray

250g green (raw) king prawns, peeled and deveined

400g boneless white fish fillets, cut into bite-size pieces

100g scallops

100g calamari, cleaned and prepared

2 cloves garlic, crushed

2 tsp chopped red chilli

1 medium red capsicum, sliced

8 shallots (spring onions), sliced

2 tbsp oyster sauce

2 tbsp fish sauce

2 tbsp water

⅓ cup shredded basil

1 Cook the rice according to the packet instructions.
2 Spray a wok or large frying pan with oil spray and place over a high heat. Cook the prawns for 1 minute, then add the fish fillets and cook for another minute. Toss in the scallops and calamari, then remove all seafood from the wok.
3 Reheat the wok and stir fry the garlic and chilli for a few seconds. Add the capsicum and shallots, and stir fry for 2–3 minutes. Add the oyster sauce, fish sauce and water, and bring to the boil. Return the seafood to the pan along with the basil and quickly toss to heat through.
4 Serve with rice.

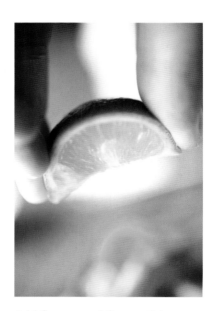

THE FOOD LOVER'S DIET

Add flavour and flare to fish, salad or veggies with a squeeze of lemon. It is a healthier choice than the salt shaker too.

Smoked salmon and corn frittata

185ml CARNATION Light & Creamy Evaporated Milk

6 large eggs

3 shallots (spring onions), thinly sliced

100g smoked salmon, coarsely shredded

1 cup corn kernels

olive or canola oil spray

1 Whisk together the evaporated milk and the eggs. Stir in the shallots, salmon and corn.

2 Spray a medium non-stick frying pan with oil spray and place over medium heat. Pour in the frittata mixture and cook slowly for approximately 5 minutes without stirring.

3 Remove from the heat and place under a preheated grill. Cook until the frittata is golden on top and completely firm.

4 Allow to stand for 1 minute before cutting into wedges and serving.

Steamed fish in foil

1 tsp sesame oil

3 tbsp lime juice

2 tbsp sweet chilli sauce

1 tbsp fish sauce

4 salmon fillets (150g each), skin removed

4 slices ginger, thinly sliced

1 stalk lemongrass, thinly sliced

3 shallots (spring onions), sliced

1 medium red capsicum, thinly sliced

1 medium carrot, cut into thin strips

500g baby bok choy, halved

fresh coriander leaves, to serve

1 Place the sesame oil, lime juice, sweet chilli sauce and fish sauce in a jug, and whisk to combine.

2 Cut four 30cm squares of aluminium foil. Place a fillet on the centre of each square of foil and top with the ginger, lemongrass and finely sliced vegetables. Fold up the edges of the foil so that none of the liquid can flow away, and then carefully pour the sauce over the fish. Loosely seal the fish in the foil, then place in a large bamboo steamer over a wok of simmering water (making sure the base of the steamer does not come into contact with the water). Cover the steamer and cook the fish in foil for 10–15 minutes, or until nearly cooked through.

3 Place the bok choy in a separate steamer on top of the fish and cook, covered, for 5 minutes, or until tender. Serve the fish parcels on top of the steamed bok choy, garnished with coriander.

A frittata is perfect when you want a meal on the table in 20 minutes. Serve it warm or cold with a salad. If you prefer, you can bake it in the oven (at 200°C for 25 minutes) in an ovenproof frying pan or pie dish.

PREP: 5 mins
COOK: 15 mins
SERVES: 4
COUNTS PER SERVE: 12

All you need to complete this meal is some rice or noodles.

PREP: 20 mins
COOK: 20 mins
SERVES: 4
COUNTS PER SERVE: 15
½ CUP COOKED RICE: 5 counts
1 CUP COOKED NOODLES: 10 counts

Like vegetables, fish is
seasonal. So ask your
fishmonger what firm
fish steaks they would
recommend you buy for
this.

PREP: 10 mins
COOK: 10 mins
SERVES: 6
COUNTS PER SERVE: 16

Stir fry fish with lemongrass and Asian greens

900g Hokkien noodles

olive or canola oil spray

500g firm fish steaks cut into large cubes

1 tsp garlic, minced

1 tsp ginger, minced

2 stalks lemongrass, finely chopped

1 medium red onion, sliced

250g baby bok choy, leaves separated

1 bunch Chinese broccoli, coarsely chopped

1 cup green capsicum, sliced

2 tbsp hoisin sauce

2 tbsp oyster sauce

1 tbsp salt-reduced soy sauce

1 tbsp rice vinegar

100g bean sprouts

1 Prepare the noodles according to the packet instructions. Drain, separate and set aside, keeping warm.

2 Spray a non-stick wok or frying pan with oil, and heat. Cook the fish in two batches over medium-high heat for 3 minutes, or until browned and tender. Set aside.

3 Reheat the wok and add the garlic, ginger, lemongrass and onion. Stir fry for 2 minutes or until soft. Add the bok choy, broccoli and capsicum, and stir fry until tender but still crisp.

4 Combine the sauces and vinegar, and stir into the wok. Return the fish to the wok and reheat.

5 Remove the stir fry from the heat and stir in the bean sprouts. Serve immediately over the noodles.

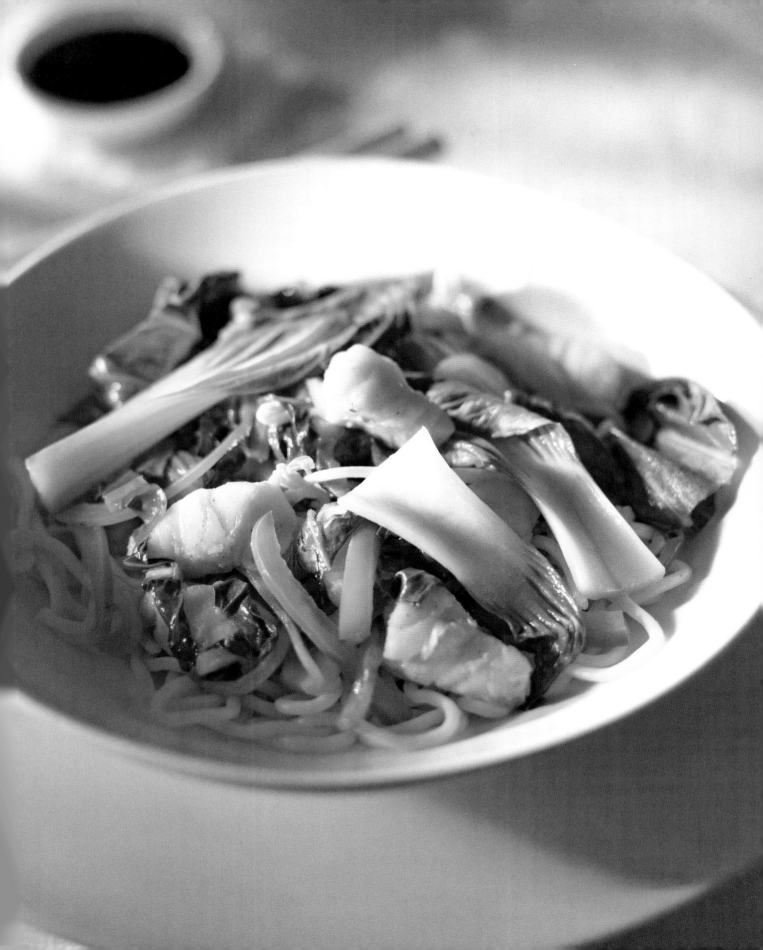

Creamy tuna pasta bake

This 'bake' is quick and easy because the filling is all prepared on the stove top and then popped under the grill to cook the cheese and heat through. You can make it with your favourite pasta shapes, such as shells or penne.

PREP: 10 mins
COOK: 15 mins
SERVES: 6
COUNTS PER SERVE: 23

400g spiral pasta

400g (or 2 x 185g) can tuna in oil, drained with 1 tbsp oil reserved

1 onion, chopped

250g button mushrooms, sliced

375ml CARNATION Light & Creamy Evaporated Milk

2 tsp wholegrain mustard

¼ cup chopped flat-leaf parsley

1 cup grated low-fat tasty cheese

1 Cook the pasta in a large saucepan according to the packet instructions. Drain and reserve the pasta.
2 While the pasta is cooking, heat the reserved tuna oil in a deep non-stick frying pan over medium heat. Add the onion and mushrooms, and cook for 4–5 minutes, or until softened and slightly browned. Add the evaporated milk and simmer for a further 2–3 minutes.
3 Preheat the grill.
4 Add the pasta, tuna, mustard and parsley to the mixture and cook for 1–2 minutes, or until warmed through.
5 Remove from the heat and transfer to four 1-cup capacity ovenproof ramekins. Sprinkle each one with some cheese, then place under the preheated grill and cook until golden brown on top. Set aside for a few minutes before serving.

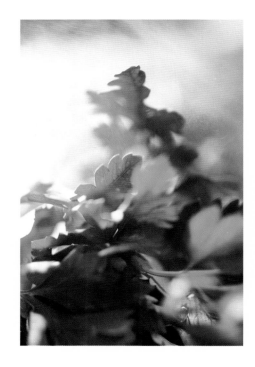

Macaroni cheese

250g macaroni

2 tsp canola or olive oil

1 medium onion, chopped

4 slices lean ham, chopped

375ml CARNATION Light & Creamy Evaporated Milk

½ cup water

1 tbsp cornflour

1 cup grated low-fat tasty cheese

2 tomatoes, sliced

½ cup wholemeal breadcrumbs

1 Cook the pasta according to the packet instructions. Drain and keep warm.
2 While the pasta is cooking, heat the oil in a pan, add the onion and cook for 2 minutes. Add the ham and cook for 1 minute.
3 Combine the evaporated milk, water and cornflour, then add to the pan and bring to the boil, stirring. Add half the cheese, then add the pasta and toss well.
4 Preheat the grill.
5 Spoon the pasta mix into a shallow ovenproof dish. Top with the tomato slices, breadcrumbs and remaining cheese. Place under a hot grill and cook until golden. Serve immediately.

Evaporated milk makes an amazingly creamy macaroni cheese without the counts you'd get using cream itself. It's a complete meal with a big green salad tossed in a vinaigrette dressing.

PREP: 15 mins
COOK: 15 mins
SERVES: 4
COUNTS PER SERVE: 27
2 CUPS SALAD TOSSED IN VINAIGRETTE
    DRESSING : 3 counts

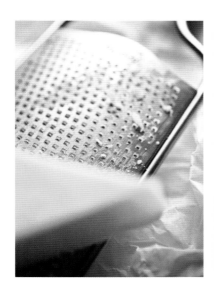

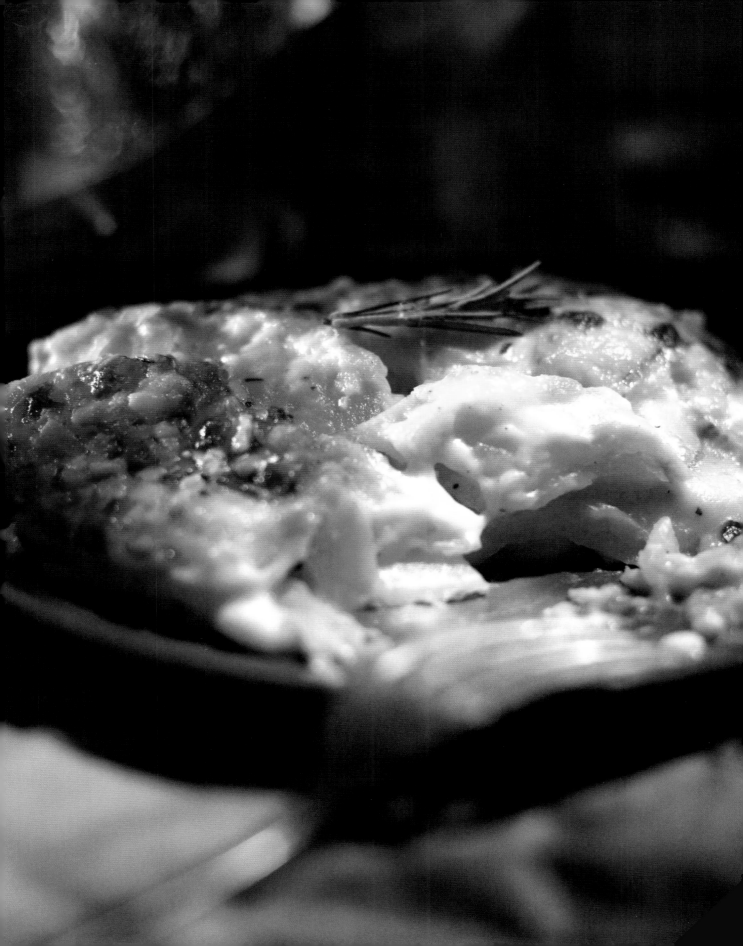

Potato bake with garlic and rosemary

60g butter or margarine

¼ cup plain flour

2⅓ cups milk

1 clove garlic, crushed

1 tsp rosemary, finely chopped

2 cups grated low-fat tasty cheese

3 large potatoes (300g each), peeled and thinly sliced

1. Preheat the oven to 180°C (160°C fan-forced). Grease a 6cm deep, 24cm square baking dish.
2. Melt the butter in a heavy-based saucepan over medium heat. Add the flour and cook, stirring constantly, for 2 minutes or until bubbly. Remove from the heat. Slowly add the milk, stirring constantly until well-combined. Return to the heat. Add the garlic and rosemary, and cook, stirring, until the sauce comes to the boil. Add 1½ cups of the cheese and stir to combine.
3. Arrange one third of the potatoes over the base of the baking dish so that they overlap slightly. Season with salt and pepper if you wish. Spoon one third of the cheese sauce over the potatoes. Repeat twice. Sprinkle the top with the remaining cheese. Bake in the oven for 1 hour, or until the potatoes are tender and the top is golden. If the top begins to brown too much, cover with foil.

Potato bake with a salad can be a meal in itself, or you can serve it as an accompaniment.

PREP: 15 mins

COOK: 1 hour 5 mins

SERVES: 4 as a meal or 6 as an accompaniment

COUNTS AS A MEAL WHEN SERVES 4: 27

COUNTS AS ACCOMPANIMENT SERVES 6: 18

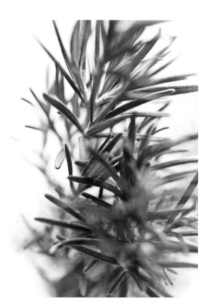

Light and creamy carbonara

Use wholemeal pasta if you want to increase your fibre intake. Serve with a salad for an extra vitamin boost, or add more vegetables to the sauce to make a complete meal. If you use the smaller (and very lean) bacon short cuts, you will need eight pieces.

PREP: 8 mins
COOK: 12 mins
SERVES: 4
COUNTS: 23

250g fettuccine

canola or olive oil spray

4 rashers rindless lean bacon, chopped

1 medium onion, chopped

2 cups mushrooms, sliced

1 cup CARNATION Light & Creamy Evaporated Milk

1 tbsp cornflour

2 tbsp grated parmesan cheese

1 Cook the pasta according to the packet instructions until al dente, then drain.

2 While the pasta is cooking, spray a non-stick frying pan with oil and place it over medium heat. Add the bacon and onion, and cook for 3 minutes, then add the mushrooms and cook for a further minute.

3 Combine the evaporated milk and cornflour, add to the pan and bring to the boil, stirring. Add the cooked pasta, then remove from the heat and sprinkle with cheese. Serve immediately.

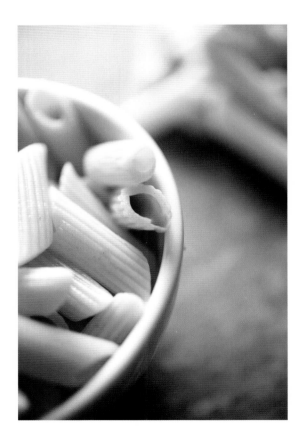

Crusty vegetable bake

1 tbsp oil

1 large onion, chopped

2 large zucchini, chopped

½ large red capsicum, chopped

1 cup chopped eggplant

60g mushrooms, sliced

410g can whole peeled tomatoes

1 packet MAGGI Cook in the Pot Chicken Cacciatore Recipe Mix

60g margarine or butter, melted

4 slices wholegrain bread, cut into squares

2 tbsp grated parmesan cheese

1 Preheat the oven to 200°C (180°C fan-forced).
2 Heat the oil in a non-stick frying pan, add the onion and cook for 2 minutes. Add the zucchini, red capsicum, eggplant and mushrooms, and cook for a further 3 minutes, stirring occasionally.
3 Combine the undrained, roughly chopped tomatoes and chicken cacciatore recipe mix, and add to the pan. Bring to the boil, stirring occasionally, then reduce the heat to low and simmer for 5 minutes. Transfer the mixture to an ovenproof casserole dish.
4 Butter the bread and spread the squares over the top of the vegetable mixture. Sprinkle with cheese and bake in the oven for 20 minutes, or until the bread is golden and crunchy.

With its crunchy, golden topping, this vegetable bake is a tasty way to get the family tucking into those much-needed vegetables.

PREP: 20 mins
COOK: 20 mins
SERVES: 4
COUNTS PER SERVE: 17

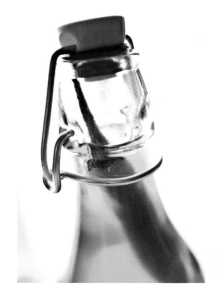

Cut back the counts with your favourite main meal recipes

It's easy. Here are some simple meal makeovers:

- ✔ Check portion sizes to make sure the recipe fits the 1, 2, 3 plate guidelines. For example, you may need to downsize the meat and potatoes portion and upsize the vegetables.
- ✔ Substitute healthier ingredients with fewer counts. For example, replace cream that's high in saturated fat with low-fat (and a healthier fat) evaporated milk.
- ✔ Reduce a higher count meal (and your housekeeping budget) by adding lower count ingredients. For example, add onion, peas and tomatoes to a frittata or lentils, or chopped celery, grated carrot and zucchini to meat sauces like chilli con carne and spaghetti bolognaise.
- ✔ Use less of the ingredients you're trying to cut back on. For example, use one rasher of bacon short cuts instead of two bacon rashers. You still get the flavour without the extra saturated fat and the added counts.

And here's how you can do it.

Meal: Meat with vegetables
- ✔ Remove the skin and trim the visible fat from the meat.
- ✔ Choose three vegetables and aim to have them take up half the plate.
- ✔ Herbs, spices or seasoning can help add taste to the meal so that everyone finishes what's on their plate.

Meal: Casserole/stew
- ✔ Choose cheaper cuts but remove the skin and trim the visible fat from the meat.
- ✔ Make it all in one pot—make sure you have protein (meat or chicken), carbohydrate (potato, pasta, etc.) and vegetables (fresh or frozen).

Meal: Roast

- Roast the meat on a wire rack over the tray and discard the fat that drains from the meat.
- Cook plenty of roast vegetables—you only need to add a small amount of oil or oil spray to get a crispy result.
- Steam, boil or microwave your beans, broccoli or cauliflower as a great side dish.

Meal: Pasta

- One cup of cooked pasta is the right amount for most of us.
- Add extra vegetables like carrots, tomato, onion and mushrooms to your sauce.
- Use a small amount of a strongly-flavoured cheese like parmesan on top—you'll need less for the same flavour.
- Replace cream with CARNATION Light & Creamy Evaporated Milk.

Meal: Salad

- You can eat as much salad as you like—it's what you toss it in and top it with that counts.
- Choose a lean protein like skinless chicken to serve with the salad.
- Dressings make a good salad taste great—use a small amount of oil with vinegar, or mustard or lemon juice.

Meal: Stir fry

- Every good stir fry has loads of fresh vegetables and a little lean meat, chicken or fish.
- Only use as much seasoning as you need to balance the flavours; no need to overdo it.
- Serve with basmati rice, or some Hokkien or rice noodles.

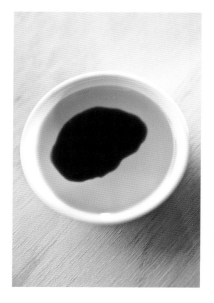

When fresh crusty bread is served with an olive oil and balsamic dipping bowl, enjoy in small quantities. Dip and count—for every dip of oil add 2 counts.

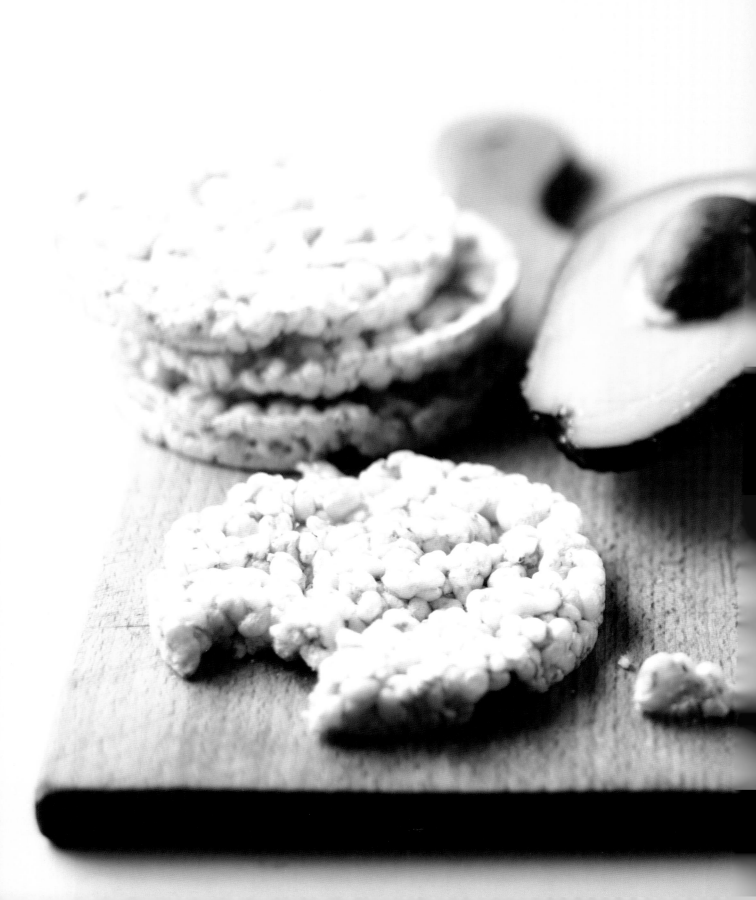

Be a guilt-free, savvy snacker. If you choose foods like fruit, vegetables, dairy foods or wholegrain cereals to snack on, you are doing something good for your health, weight and your energy levels. Snacks like these give you a 'nutrient kick', upping your intake of vitamins, minerals, calcium and fibre. In fact, if you just eat three meals a day it can be hard to hit your daily targets for fruit (two serves), vegetables (five serves) and dairy foods (three serves), which is why the right snack at the right time can do wonders for your wellbeing.

The food lover's way to healthy snacking

Give your brain a boost and improve your alertness and concentration.

Stop hunger in its tracks. You'll eat less at your next meal. It's true—the flow-on effect of healthy snacking is that you don't over-eat at the next meal, and you'll be less likely to bolt your food.

It's good to remember: Healthy snacks can provide essential nutrients. A good snack will be around 4 to 7 counts once or twice a day, or as best suits you and your routine.

Sustain your energy levels and get through that long 'to do' list.

Q&A

Q: I am definitely one of those people who needs to eat several smaller meals a day. Can you give me some 'snack-attack' tips?

A: First of all, don't snack if you're not hungry—it shouldn't be a way of filling in time when you're bored, or trying to cheer yourself up. Here's what we find helpful:

- Keep water on hand. Thirst can be mistaken for hunger, so have a glass of water before you eat something and see if you're still hungry 20 minutes later.
- If it's healthy, keep it handy. Keep nuts, seeds, dried fruit, single-serve tubs of fruit or yoghurt, wholegrain crackers, packet soups, popcorn, baked beans and canned fish on hand. Keep a loaf of bread in the freezer—that way you can just pop a piece in the toaster when you need a quick fix.
- Watch that portion size—snacks should generally be no more than 7 counts.

Q: What's the difference between snacks and treats?

A: *Snacking* isn't about eating more food; it's about spreading the same amount of food over more frequent, smaller meals. Depending on what you eat, snacks can make a significant contribution to a healthy diet, providing important nutrients. In this chapter we give you ideas for plenty of snacks that only cost around 7 counts.

Treats are extras (and quite often come with double-figure counts). Although delicious (and most of us love them), they generally don't provide us with the essential nutrients our bodies need. On top of that, they are often made with too much fat, salt or sugar. So think of treats as occasional foods and keep them for, well, a treat. Savour treats by indulging in a small amount of something you really enjoy, or share treats with a friend and just have half.

Q: I get hunger pangs at 4 p.m. What's a healthy snack to get me through to dinnertime without reaching for the cookie jar?

A: We often suggest a 'diet' yoghurt in these circumstances. They are low in fat and sugars, and so don't have many counts. They come in a range of flavours, so you shouldn't get bored. Try keeping a week's supply in the fridge at work (write your name on the top in big black letters as they tend to disappear). When you get those hunger pangs, you can eat one at your desk while working. They don't leave any crumbs, so you won't look unprofessional. Remember to wash the spoon!

Drinking juice is just as good as eating fruit

No. Drinking juice isn't the same as eating fresh fruit at all. First of all, you are missing out on the fibre—for example, home-squeezed orange juice has only a quarter of the fibre you'd get if you ate the orange instead, which is one reason it will leave you feeling less full. On top of that, even a small glass of juice will have twice the number of counts as a fresh orange because it's concentrated. It takes two or three oranges to fill that little 200ml (¾ cup) glass.

Banana bread is a healthy type of bread

Banana bread is actually cake (and so are muffins). A typical slice of banana bread will have you notching up 9 or more counts, and that's without adding on toppings like jam and ricotta or margarine.

It says it's natural on the label, so it's better for me

No. Just because a food is from natural sources doesn't mean it will always be better for you. Butter and full-cream milk are 'natural', but they still contain lots of saturated fat.

It's a good choice because it's in the health food aisle

Not necessarily. The health food aisle or health or organic food shops don't always have a health halo hovering overhead. Many snack foods stacked on the 'health food' shelves are way too high in salt (sodium), fat (including saturated fat) and sugar, which can really notch up the counts without doing anything for your health. Some of the products are just designed for people who have a specific dietary requirement—like gluten free—and don't really have anything to do with the product itself being healthy.

If it's baked, not fried, it's a better option

Not always. Salty biscuits and chips might claim they are baked, but if they use the same amount of fat to bake or fry the food, they'll have just as many counts. So always check the nutrition information before making your choice.

Nuts are fattening

Not if you choose the unsalted, raw or dry-roasted varieties, and stick to a small handful a day—which, as a guide, is about 20 almonds or 15 cashews. Many people avoid nuts, for fear they will stack on the kilos. However, nuts are actually a great source of healthy fats and are very satiating. Just a small handful a day may help reduce your blood cholesterol.

Myth
buster

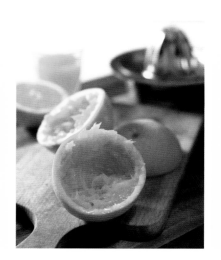

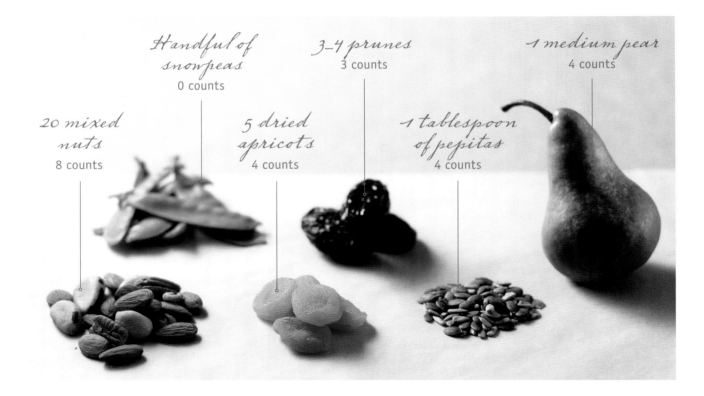

Handful of snowpeas
0 counts

3–4 prunes
3 counts

1 medium pear
4 counts

20 mixed nuts
8 counts

5 dried apricots
4 counts

1 tablespoon of pepitas
4 counts

Smart snacks

A piece of fresh fruit. It's sweet, portable and comes ready wrapped in its own packaging. Choose fruits in season to add variety.

A single-serve (shelf-stable) tub of fruit salad or diced fruit is a great alternative to have on hand in the cupboard (or desk drawer).

Dried fruits keep well and don't squash, but keep portions small as they are a very concentrated source of counts.

Carrot and celery sticks, snow peas or a few crispy beans. Crunch away, or dunk into a dip like low-fat hummus or tzatziki.

A cup of vegetable soup, like pumpkin, tomato, lentil or minestrone, is a great way to pack extra vegetables into your day.

A slice of grainy bread or grainy toast, or a couple of grainy crackers or wholegrain crispbreads make a quick and easy snack topped with a smear of Vegemite or peanut butter, some sliced tomato, cottage cheese, or a little jam or honey if you want something sweet.

Unsalted nuts (just a small handful)—make your own nut and seed mix by mixing equal amounts of cashews, almonds, peanuts, pumpkin seeds and sunflower seeds.

A hard-boiled egg, or a small can of tuna, salmon or sardines pack in some protein power.

A small tub of reduced-fat yoghurt, or a fromage frais dairy dessert like Frûche, a slice of cheese or a small carton of milk (flavoured is OK) deliciously ups your healthy dairy intake. Warning! Don't be fooled into thinking the yoghurt you buy in the fruit shop is automatically low in fat. Most fruit shop yoghurts actually have cream added to them, which is why they taste so … creamy! Double check the ingredients list next time. And if the tub doesn't have an ingredients list on it, don't buy it.

SNACK MATHS: TEN EVERYDAY SNACK COMBOS WITH NO MORE THAN 7 COUNTS

A 200g tub of diet vanilla yoghurt (4)	+ 3 large sliced strawberries (2)	+ a small handful of blueberries (1)	7
2 wholegrain crackers (2)	+ 1 thick (30g) slice of 25% reduced-fat cheese (5)	+ 2 slices of tomato, with pepper to taste (0)	7
Blend together ½ cup skim milk (2)	+ ½ a 200g tub of diet banana yoghurt (2)	+ ½ a medium banana (3)	7
Chop 1 small carrot into sticks (2)	+ 3 stalks of celery cut into sticks (0)	+ ⅓ cup of tzatziki for dipping (3)	5
4 rye crackers (2)	+ a small 95g can of 98% fat-free tomato and onion tuna in water, drained (4)		6
A slice of toasted light fruit loaf (4)	+ 2 tbsp of ricotta cheese (3)		7
A thin slice of toasted multigrain bread (3)	+ 1 heaped tsp of peanut butter (3)		6
4 slices of fresh pear (2)	+ 4 tsp of reduced-fat cottage cheese (2)	+ 4 walnut halves (2)	6
1 cup of packet tomato soup (4)	+ a piece of toasted wholemeal bread (3)		7
2 rice crackers (1)	+ 2 tsp of light cream cheese (1)	+ 2 tsp of fruit conserve or jam (2)	4

Snack on dairy foods

The dairy aisle can be confusing, but here's how you can cut to the chase and make smart choices.

Priority # 1: Reduced fat

Make reduced-fat dairy foods your top priority most of the time—reduced-fat or skim milks, low-fat or no-fat yoghurts, and reduced-fat dairy desserts, custard, ice cream and cheese. These products are also fine for children over the age of two. By cutting back the fat, you slash the counts. In fact, skim milk has just over half the number of counts as full-cream milk. So, how much fat is in that milk?

- **Regular milk** (full cream or whole milk) on average contains 3.8% milk fat and no less than 3.2% milk fat—1 cup = 8 counts.
- **Reduced-fat milk** has approximately 2% milk fat and it may have extra protein and calcium added—1 cup = 7 counts.
- **Low-fat milk** has less than 1.5% milk fat and similar nutritional benefits—1 cup = 6 counts.
- **Skim milk** has no more than 0.15% milk fat. Milk solids are added for optimum taste—1 cup = 5 counts.

Priority # 2: Calcium bonus

Milk is an important source of calcium for most of us. To get that 1000mg plus of calcium a day for strong bones, it's recommended we have three serves of dairy foods. It's not hard. Here's what a serve of dairy food looks like:

- ✔ 1 cup (250ml) milk—choose reduced fat.
- ✔ 1 cup (250ml) calcium-enriched soy milk—choose reduced fat.
- ✔ 1 cup (200ml) low-fat yoghurt or calcium-enriched soy yoghurt.
- ✔ 40g hard cheese (about 2 slices)—use reduced-fat varieties most often.
- ✔ ⅓ cup shredded cheese—use reduced-fat varieties most often.
- ✔ ½ cup (125ml) skim or reduced-fat evaporated milk.

Cheese choices

- Opt for reduced-fat cheese where there's a choice.
- Cheeses that have been 'matured' for a longer time, like cheddar cheese, have a higher calcium content than 'unripened' cheeses like cottage and ricotta cheese.
- Keep cheeses like brie and camembert for special occasions. Think of them as treat foods.

Can't have dairy?

Don't be dismayed. There are some great soy alternatives on the supermarket shelves, but just make sure they are reduced fat and **calcium fortified** to ensure they're building your bones, too. Other non-dairy options that will boost your calcium intake include: almonds, brazil nuts, sesame seeds, dried figs, tinned fish, dark leafy greens, dried beans including soybeans, calcium-enriched tofu and calcium-fortified breakfast cereals like UNCLE TOBYS PLUS cereals range.

Simple snacks for all occasions

Choose portion-controlled snacks or make up your own combos from the following foods, and count your way to a healthy life and weight. The counts we give here are only average counts for these typical foods. If you check out the ready-reckoner, you can find the counts for your favourite products.

Typical counts for breads, cereals and crackers

- **1 count** = three wholegrain rice crackers; a multigrain corn thin; a rye cruskit; a wholegrain wheat cracker (Vita-Weat).
- **3 counts** = 2 cups of air-popped popcorn.
- **4 counts** = a thin slice of multigrain, wholemeal or white bread, or fruit loaf; a crumpet; half an English muffin.
- **5 counts** = a small bag of cereal (CHEERIOS).
- **6 counts** = a wholegrain cereal bar; a small bag of cereal bites (Fruity Bites).
- **7 counts** = a bowl of wholegrain cereal such as WEETIES with skim milk.

Toppings

- **2 counts** = 1 teaspoon of margarine, peanut butter, jam or honey; 1 tablespoon of reduced-fat ricotta or low-fat cottage cheese; 2 slices of avocado or 1 tablespoon of hummus.

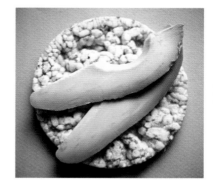

A thick rice cake with avocado is a great snack for only 4 counts.

Typical counts for dairy foods, eggs, canned fish, legumes, or nuts and seeds

- **4 counts** = a 200g tub of 'diet' yoghurt; 100g of reduced-fat custard; one medium hard-boiled egg; one small can of flavoured tuna or salmon (in water, drained) in a lettuce cup; two scoops of no-added-sugar and calcium-fortified ice cream.
- **5 counts** = a regular size skinny latte or cappuccino; a 125g tub of low-fat fromage frais; 1 cup (250ml) of reduced-fat soy milk; two slices of extra-light cheddar cheese; a small single-serve can of baked beans in tomato sauce.
- **6 counts** = 1 cup (250ml) of reduced-fat milk; 2 teaspoons of MILO with a small glass of skim milk; 3 teaspoons of NESQUIK with a small glass of skim milk; a small handful (20g) of unsalted, roasted nuts or nut and seed mix.

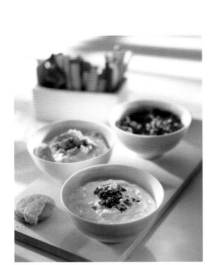

Typical counts for fruit and vegetables

- **Free** = celery and carrot sticks; tiny tomatoes; capsicum slices; blanched snow peas; cauliflower florets; canned asparagus spears; button mushrooms.
- **2 counts** = one medium mandarin; half a medium pawpaw; two large apricots.
- **3 counts** = one medium kiwifruit; one large peach or nectarine; two medium plums; one (3cm) thick slice of watermelon; ½ tablespoon of sultanas; four dried apricots; ten dried apple rings; four dates.
- **4 counts** = 1 cup of fresh fruit salad; one medium apple; one small banana; one medium orange; one medium pear; a small bunch (22) of grapes; one small glass (200ml/¾ cup) of fruit juice.

Dip it!

- **2 counts** = 1 tablespoon of hummus or French onion dip; 2 tablespoons of tzatziki or beetroot dip; 4 tablespoons of tomato salsa.

Savvy snacking

It's the way we snack that can be the problem—what we choose, when we have it and why we're eating it. So let's troubleshoot some snack-attack issues:

Problem: The kitchen cupboard is calling …

Solution: Think of your kitchen as a café with a closing time, after which food is no longer served. After any meal, tidy up, and turn off the lights. That way you'll be less tempted to return.

Problem: Mindless snacking for any reason other than real hunger.

Solution: First of all, be aware of your 'snack-attack' triggers—watching TV, or at the supermarket checkout. Secondly, be prepared. Keep water and healthy snacks on hand, and save yourself from impulse purchases.

Problem: The afternoon munchies have hit and the vending machine is near …

Solution: Be prepared and plan ahead to avoid getting into this situation. Fill your desk drawer with snacks, like wholegrain cereal bars, packet vegetable soups and nuts, for when you need them.

Count the difference with snacks

CHOOSE THIS …	NOT THIS
Fruit Loaf (30g) + thin spread margarine = 6 counts	Banana bread (60g slice) + thin spread margarine = 11 counts
Mini wholegrain biscuits (17 biscuits, or 20g) = 4 counts	1 mini packet (about 10) Shape biscuits = 6 counts
1 fresh orange = 3 counts	Small bottle orange juice (300ml) = 6 counts
Wholegrain muesli bar = 6 counts	Medium muffin = 10 counts
Diet (no fat or sugar) yoghurt (200g tub) = 4 counts	Regular yoghurt (200g tub) = 10 counts
Air-popped popcorn (2 cups) = 3 counts	Potato chips (30g packet) = 6 counts
Lite hummus dip (2 tbsp) = 3 counts	Regular hummus dip (2 tbsp) = 5 counts
Wasabi peas (¼ cup) = 6 counts	10 pretzels = 11 counts
2 pikelets with jam = 5 counts	Doughnut = 11 counts
4 wholegrain rice crackers = 1 count	4 Jatz crackers = 3 counts
2 slices extra-light cheddar cheese (50% less fat) = 5 counts	2 slices regular cheddar cheese = 8 counts

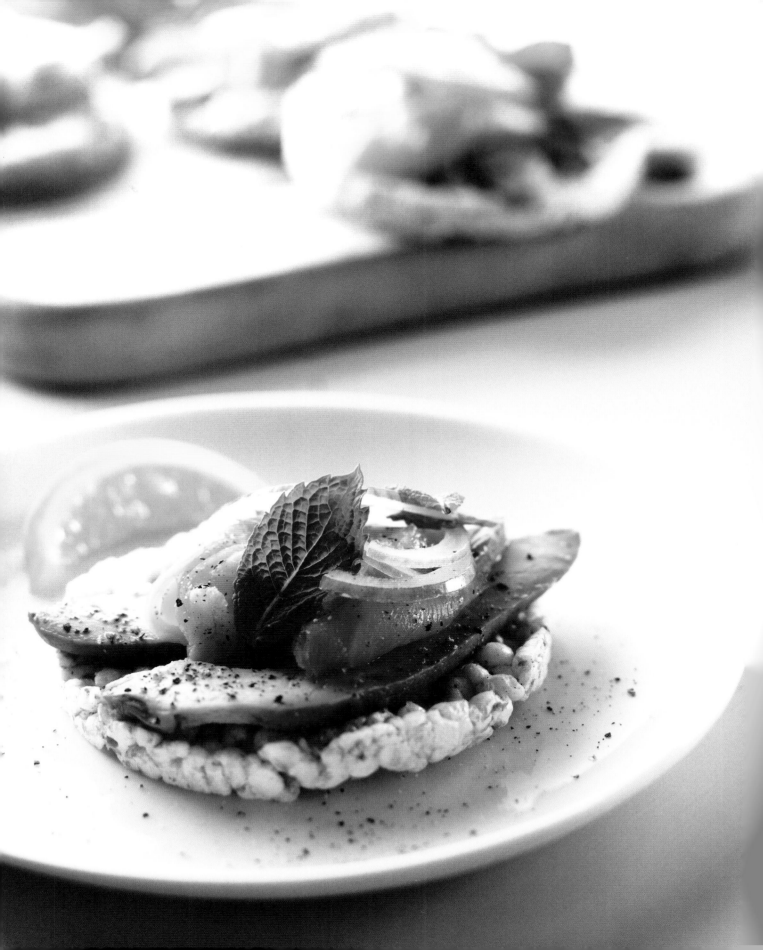

Healthy snack recipes

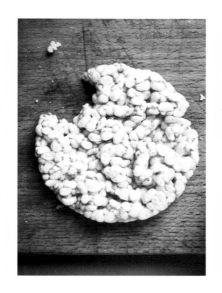

Rice cakes with egg and hummus

4 thick rice cakes

4 tbsp hummus

1 tbsp chopped flat-leaf parsley leaves

2 hard-boiled eggs, peeled and sliced

¼ tsp smoked paprika

freshly ground black pepper

1 Spread each rice cake with 1 tablespoon of hummus, sprinkle with chopped parsley and top with egg. Season with paprika and pepper.

Rice cakes make a good snack at only 2 counts each. If you prefer, pop these tasty toppings on toast, multigrain crackers or rye crispbread.

PREP: 5 mins
MAKES: 4
COUNTS PER SERVE: 6

Rice cakes with smoked fish and avocado

4 thick rice cakes

1 small avocado, peeled and sliced

100g smoked fish, such as salmon or trout

½ small red onion, peeled and finely sliced

fresh mint leaves

1 Top each rice cake with avocado before piling on the fish, onion and mint leaves.

Add colour, texture and taste with toppings to satisfy all your senses.

PREP: 5 mins
MAKES: 4
COUNTS PER SERVE: 9

PREP: 5 mins
MAKES: 4
COUNTS PER SERVE: 8

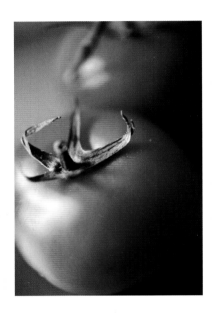

PREP: 5 mins
MAKES: 4
COUNTS PER SERVE: 4

Rice cakes with pastrami and tomato

4 thick rice cakes

4 slices pastrami

8 tbsp reduced-fat cottage cheese

2 tomatoes, sliced

4 fresh basil leaves

freshly ground black pepper

1 Top each rice cake with a slice of pastrami, 2 tablespoons of cottage cheese, a few slices of tomato and a basil leaf. Season with freshly ground black pepper.

Rice cakes with beef and horseradish 'mayo'

2 tbsp mayonnaise

½–1 tsp prepared horseradish, to taste

4 thick rice cakes

4 slices 'deli' roast beef

1 Combine mayonnaise with prepared horseradish to taste.
2 Place a slice of beef on each rice cake and top with horseradish mayo.

Pumpkin and roasted garlic hummus

1 small red onion, peeled and chopped

300g can chickpeas, drained

250g can NESTLÉ Reduced Cream

1 packet pumpkin and roasted garlic soup mix

1 tbsp lemon juice

1 Place the onion and chickpeas in a food processor or blender and pulse until smooth. Shake can of reduced cream then open, combine with soup mix and add to chickpeas in the food processor, together with the lemon juice. Pulse until the dip is creamy smooth.

2 Spoon into a bowl, cover and chill for 30 minutes before serving.

If you want a creamy dip, you can have it. How? Choose a reduced-fat cream like this (which is 25% fat compared with regular cream at 35% fat) and keep an eye on portion size—it's still 3 counts per tablespoon.

PREP: 5 mins
CHILL: 30 mins
MAKES: 1½ cups
COUNTS (PER 1 TBSP): 3

Feta and rosemary dip with pita crisps

250g can NESTLÉ Reduced Cream

100g reduced-fat feta cheese

2 tsp fresh rosemary, chopped

1 tsp lemon juice

½ tsp lemon zest

1 packet wholemeal pita rounds

olive oil spray

1 Shake can of reduced cream, open and pour into a bowl. Crumble in the feta. Add the rosemary, lemon juice and zest, and mix well to a creamy consistency. Cover and chill for 30 minutes before serving with pita rounds.

2 Alternatively, to make your own pita crisps, cut large wholemeal pita rounds into eight wedges and pull the wedges apart to make two triangles. Spread on a baking tray lined with baking paper, spray lightly with olive oil spray and bake in a preheated oven at 180°C (160°C fan-forced) for 10–15 minutes until crisp.

Dips are a great way to add flavour to steamed or boiled vegetables.

PREP: 5 mins
CHILL: 30 mins
MAKES: 1 cup
COUNTS (PER 1 TBSP): 3
PITA CRISPS: Add 1 count for 2 crisps

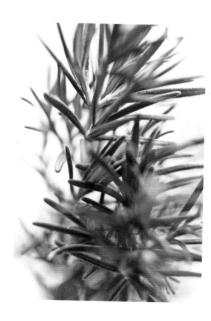

This pretty, pale green dip
is delicious with crudités
for easy entertaining and
snacks.

PREP: 5 mins
CHILL: 30 mins
MAKES: 1½ cups
COUNTS (PER 1 TBSP): 2

Pea, mint and feta dip

250g can NESTLÉ Reduced Cream

1 packet onion soup mix

100g reduced-fat feta cheese

¼ cup fresh mint leaves, finely chopped

1 cup peas, cooked, drained and cooled

2 tsp lemon juice

1 Shake can of reduced cream, open and pour into food processor
   or blender. Add remaining ingredients, and pulse until creamy and
   smooth.
2 Cover and chill for 30 minutes before serving.

Fruit bread toast toppers

For 7 counts, toast a slice of dense fruit bread and top with:

- 2 tbsp low-fat ricotta and a sprinkle of cinnamon.
- 1 tbsp low-fat cottage cheese and 2 tsp 100% berry spread.
- Half a small banana, mashed, and a drizzle of maple syrup.

Freshly baked scones
are always popular when
friends or family visit. If
you make them gluten free
it's much more inclusive as
these days there's bound to
be someone who prefers or
needs to avoid gluten for
health reasons.

PREP: 10 mins
CHILL: 25 mins
MAKES: 16
COUNTS PER SERVE: 7

Gluten-free cheese and chive scones

2½ cups gluten-free self-raising flour

2 packets MAGGI Gluten Free Tasty Cheese Sauce Mix

1 tbsp chopped chives, optional

375g CARNATION Light & Creamy Evaporated Milk

15g butter or margarine, melted

⅓ cup grated tasty cheese

1 Preheat the oven to 220°C (200°C fan-forced). Lightly grease a
   baking tray.
2 Sift the flour into a bowl, then add cheese sauce mix and chives. Stir
   in the evaporated milk until well-combined and the dough is sticky.
3 Knead the dough on a well-floured surface until smooth. Pat the
   dough to 2cm thickness and cut out scones using a floured 5cm
   round cutter.
4 Place the scones side by side on the prepared tray, brush the tops
   with butter and sprinkle with grated tasty cheese. Bake in the oven
   for 20–25 minutes until golden.

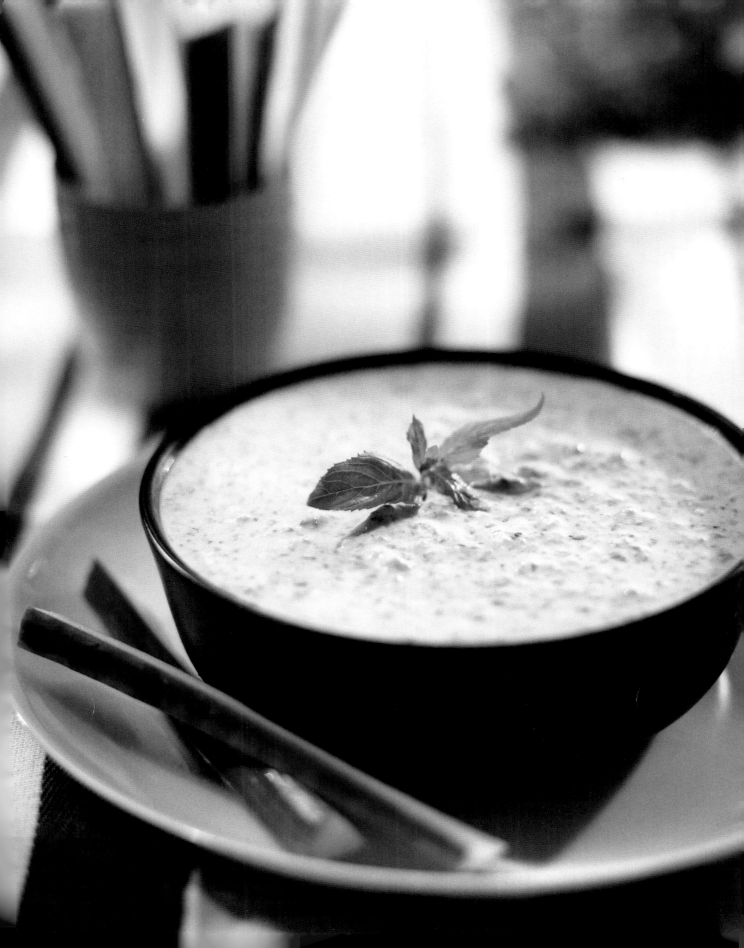

PREP: 20 mins
COOK: 12 mins
MAKES: 40
COUNTS PER PIECE: 3

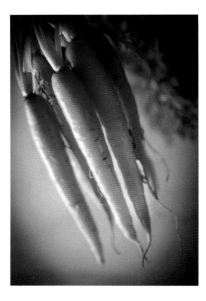

Bakes like this make great snacks. Enjoy as a light meal first and pop the leftovers into your lunch box.

PREP: 10 mins
CHILL: 25 mins
SERVES: 4
COUNTS PER SERVE: 9

Savoury cheese twisters

2½ cups wholemeal plain flour

1 tsp mustard powder

125g margarine

1 cup grated light tasty cheese

250ml CARNATION Light & Creamy Evaporated Milk

3 tbsp Vegemite or Marmite

1 Preheat oven to 200°C (180°C fan-forced) and line two oven trays with baking paper.
2 Sift flour and mustard powder in a large bowl. Rub in margarine until the mixture resembles breadcrumbs and stir in the cheese. Add evaporated milk and mix to form dough.
3 Roll the dough out on a lightly floured surface to form a rectangle approximately 25cm x 45cm, then spread Vegemite over the dough.
4 Fold the dough in half, then roll it up and cut it into two. Cut forty 1½ cm strips. Twist the strips, place on prepared trays and bake for 12 minutes, or until golden. Cool on a wire rack.

Carrot and zucchini bake

1 packet MAGGI 99% fat free 2 Minute Noodles Chicken Flavour

2 eggs

½ cup low-fat milk

1 pinch ground nutmeg

1 medium zucchini, grated

1 medium carrot, grated

½ cup grated gruyére cheese

1 Preheat the oven to 180°C. Line a 20cm round cake tin with baking paper.
2 Break the noodle cake into eight pieces. In a bowl beat together the eggs, milk, nutmeg and flavour sachet. Add the noodles, zucchini, carrot and cheese, then mix to combine.
3 Spoon the mixture into the prepared tin and bake for 25 minutes. Turn the bake out of the tin and serve cold.

Dried fruit and sunflower seed muffin bars

¾ cup dried mixed fruit

½ cup water

400g skim sweetened condensed milk

½ cup skim milk

1 cup self-raising flour, sifted

1 cup traditional rolled oats

½ cup sunflower seeds

1 Preheat the oven to 180°C (160°C fan-forced). Grease and line an 18cm x 28cm lamington tin with baking paper.
2 Place the dried fruit and water in a medium saucepan and bring to the boil. Simmer gently until the liquid is absorbed. Remove from the heat. Add the condensed milk and skim milk to the dried fruit mixture, then set aside.
3 In a large bowl, mix together the flour, oats and sunflower seeds. Stir the wet ingredients into the flour mixture and mix thoroughly before pressing the mixture into the prepared tin.
4 Bake for 20 minutes, or until golden and cooked through when tested with a skewer. While still warm cut into fourteen bars.

Packed with goodies like seeds, oats and dried fruit, these muffin bars make a dense and chewy snack that's sure to keep the hunger pangs at bay.

PREP: 10 mins
COOK: 20 mins
MAKES: 14
COUNTS PER SERVE: 9

Asian chicken and corn noodle soup

Packet soups are perfect for a more substantial snack, but this recipe shows you how easy it is to make your own super tasty soup from scratch.

PREP: 5 mins
COOK: 5 mins
SERVES: 4
COUNTS PER SERVE: 11

2 packets MAGGI 2 Minute Noodles Chicken Flavour

5 cups boiling water

1 tbsp soy sauce

¼ tsp ginger puree

2 tsp brown sugar

420g can corn kernels, drained

¼ cooked chicken, skin and bones removed, shredded

1 shallot (spring onion), sliced thinly

¼ cup coriander leaves

1 Break the noodle cakes into quarters. In a pan combine the noodles, contents of flavour sachets, water, soy sauce, ginger, brown sugar and corn kernels. Bring to the boil and simmer for 2 minutes. Stir in the remaining ingredients and serve immediately.

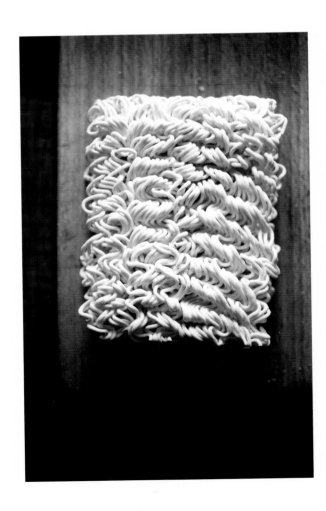

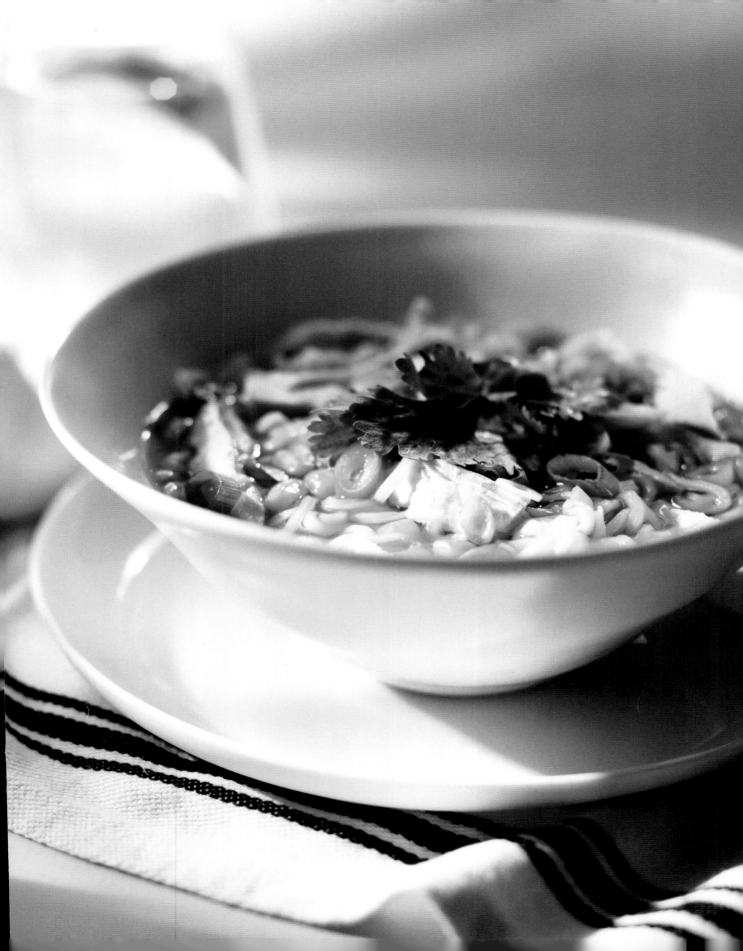

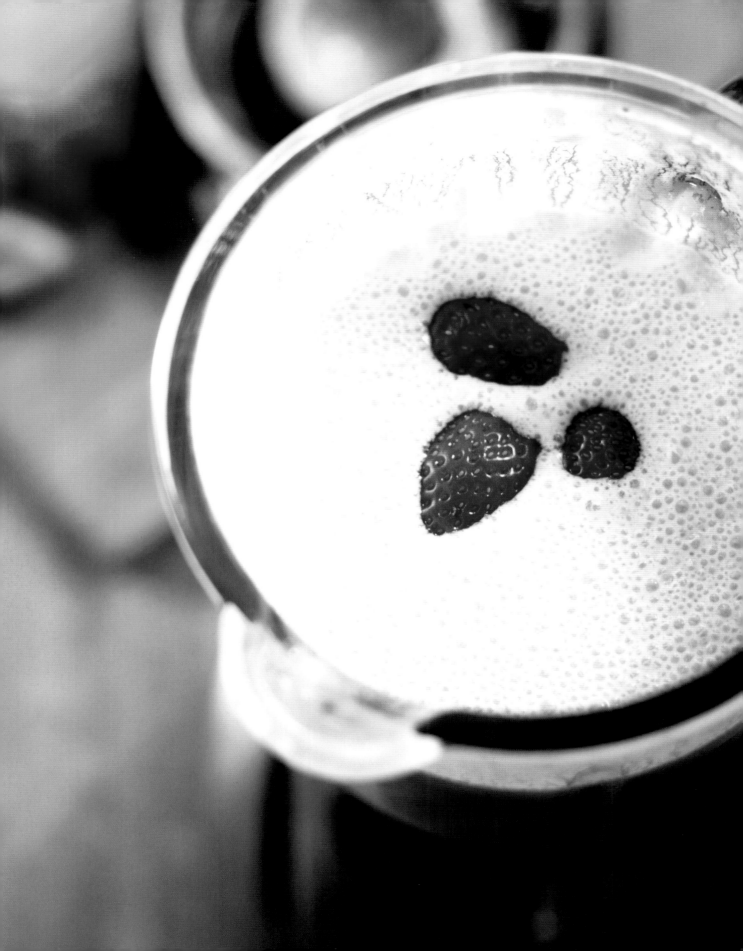

We all know the best drink in the world for quenching our thirst and keeping us hydrated is cool, clear water. It's essential for life and it's free. But these days we are spoilt for choice when it comes to beverages—there are drinks for when we are active, drinks for resting and relaxing, party drinks, special drinks for extra energy, drinks for better skin, drinks with more vitamins, extra antioxidants, and so the list goes on. So if we think before we drink, we can achieve a happy life and weight by keeping some counts for the drinks we really love.

Drinks for food lovers

Tea and coffee are enjoyed all over the world as drinks to stimulate, recharge or refresh us.

Milk (especially low-fat) is a great way to get the calcium needed to build and maintain healthy bones.

Water is essential for life. We can live without food for weeks, but only days without water.

All fluids count towards our daily need for 8–10 cups, including coffee and tea.

Take care with what you drink. Some drinks are more like mini meals, giving you more counts than you want.

It's good to remember: Drinks can provide 0 counts to a huge 25 or more counts a day depending on your choices. Consider 'high count' drinks that are low in nutrition as a treat, keeping them to 10 counts per day if you choose to drink them.

Q&A

Q: I feel tired and headachy in the afternoon and a colleague said it is because I am probably dehydrated. Do you think that's the case?

A: If you are constantly tired and headachy, it's probably a good idea to see your doctor. But dehydration is much more common than you might imagine. Many of us are now coming to realise that having a bottle of water on our desk that reminds us to drink during the day is a good thing—especially if the water cooler is at the other end of the office. I just use filtered tap water in mine and refill it first thing each morning when I arrive at work. Tea, coffee and herbal teas are also useful sources of fluid and help you to stay hydrated, and they add a bit of variety.

It's good to remember:
Drink counts can add up to a meal size.

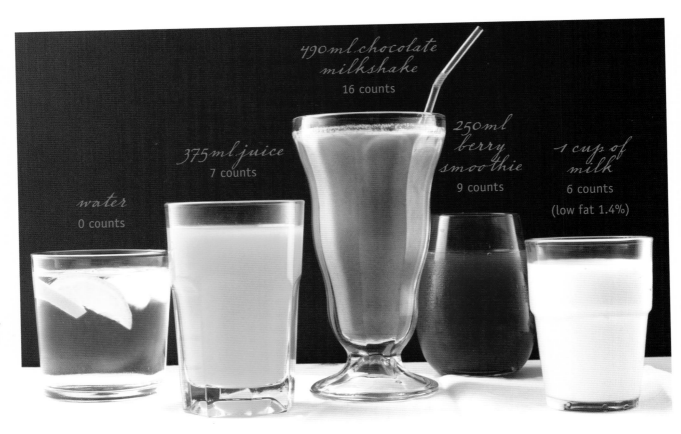

490ml chocolate milkshake
16 counts

375ml juice
7 counts

250ml berry smoothie
9 counts

1 cup of milk
6 counts
(low fat 1.4%)

water
0 counts

Myth buster

Coffee and tea are dehydrating

No, not in moderation. It is well known that caffeine found in coffee and tea (as well as other drinks such as energy drinks) can cause an initial mild diuretic effect, which means they cause the body to lose more water from the kidneys. However, this has been found to diminish over time with regular consumption. Regularly drinking caffeine-containing beverages such as coffee and tea does not cause dehydration, and in fact does contribute to your daily fluid requirements.

Instant coffee is bad for you

No. Instant coffee contains no additives and is simply brewed coffee beans that have had the water removed to produce coffee granules or powder. In terms of caffeine, it has been shown that 300–400mg of caffeine a day is safe and associated with coffee's beneficial effects of boosting energy, alertness and concentration. In instant coffee terms, that's equivalent to 3–4 cups.

Low-carb beers help lose weight

Not necessarily. It's the kilojoules that count, not the carbs. Low-carb beers are in fact not that much lower in counts than regular beers as they are still high in alcohol.

We need eight glasses of water a day

It's fluid we need—it doesn't have to be just plain water. All drinks and many foods (especially fruit and vegetables) contain water. As we get about a quarter of our water needs from food, we need to consume about 8–10 cups of fluid (from all drinks) each day to replace what we lose through our skin, intestines and kidneys. We should get **most** of this from plain water (whether it's tap, filtered or bottled) as it's free (no counts), but other drinks in moderation can be included for variety, enjoyment and even some added nutritional value.

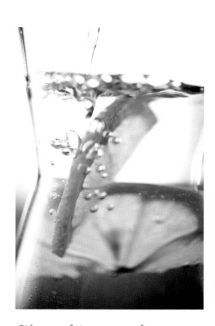

It's good to remember: Add a slice of lemon to chilled water for a refreshing drink that has no added sugar and no counts. Its one of life's simple pleasures.

Water for life

Water keeps our blood flowing, regulates our body temperature, and assists in digestion and flushing out toxins. In the short term, dehydration leads to thirst, fatigue and irritability. A lack of concentration is often due to not being well hydrated. If tap water isn't your thing, try soda or mineral water, or even popping in a slice of lemon or lime for some extra zing. An investment in a water filter may be worthwhile as it can improve the taste. Chilling water can also make it easier to drink.

Keeping the kids hydrated

What our kids drink is important for their overall health. If we can teach them good drinking habits and guide them to make good drink choices, then we set them up for better health in the long term. Like us, they should avoid high-count drinks that provide little other nutrients—particularly fizzy drinks, cordials and fruit drinks, which are not good for their teeth, can displace other more nutritious drinks or can contribute to unhealthy weight gain. These are best kept for special events. Nutritionists and dentists advise us that our kids' fluid needs are best met with water and milk. Water should be what they are given in their drink bottles, and they should be encouraged to drink regularly, particularly in hot weather, as kids are more prone to dehydration than adults.

Coffee and tea

Coffee and tea are both rich in antioxidants, which are thought to help keep our bodies healthy. The caffeine content is what helps boost our alertness and concentration. For some people it can have unwanted effects, but this is generally at high levels. Unsweetened coffee and tea, even with a little milk, provide less than 1 count per serve. Be wary of café coffees made with full-cream milk, though, as the counts are much higher. This table shows how the counts stack up according to how you have your coffee or tea.

It's good to remember: Don't sip continuously. Your saliva needs time to return your mouth to a healthy pH environment to prevent dental caries.

Tea with skim milk	Tea bag = 0	²⁄₃ cup (170ml) hot water = 0	1½ tbsp (30ml) skim milk = 1	1
Skinny coffee	1 tsp NESCAFÉ coffee = 0	²⁄₃ cup (170ml) hot water = 0	1½ tbsp (30ml) skim milk = 1	1
Chai tea	½ cup (125ml) water = 0	Chai tea = 0	½ cup (125ml) regular milk = 4	4
Skinny latte	Espresso coffee = 0	¾ cup (200ml) skim milk = 4	Equal sweetener = 0	4
Regular latte and sugar	Espresso coffee = 0	¾ cup (200ml) regular milk = 6	1 tsp sugar = 1	7
Regular mocha	Espresso coffee = 0	¾ cup (200ml) regular milk = 6	1 tbsp chocolate syrup = 3	9

Milk and milk drinks

Milk is rich in essential nutrients, including protein and calcium. Choose reduced-fat milk in preference to full-cream milk, which is high in saturated fat. Toddlers under two years of age should be given whole milk only because they are growing rapidly and need fat to provide the energy for growth and development. Although milk does contain a natural sugar, it also has other tooth-friendly nutrients, so it is safer on teeth between meals.

Flavoured milk is milk with added sugar and extra counts. Although plain milk is best, flavoured milk is better than no milk at all. Some options also contain additional vitamins and minerals, which make them an even more nourishing source of energy. Be wary of the ready-to-drink flavoured milks in cartons or bottles, often sold in convenience stores—the serve sizes can be huge (500 or 600ml), with one bottle providing up to 20 counts. These are more of a meal than a snack, so drink them sparingly.

Soy, rice and oat 'milk' drinks are alternatives to cow's milk, but it is essential to choose ones that are fortified with calcium. If you are watching your weight, you should choose the light option—calcium enriched, of course, too.

Smoothies and shakes

Made with milk and fruit, smoothies are mainly full of things good for your health, and they're an easy snack when you are at home. They can, however, contain added sugar, honey or even ice cream—particularly those bought in cafés—thereby massively increasing the counts they deliver. You should think of juice bar smoothies as more like a meal, and ideally choose low-fat milk and go for the small serve size.

MILK DRINK MATHS

Skinny shake	1 cup (250ml) skim milk = 5	3 tbsp diet chocolate syrup = 1			6
Flavoured milk	¾ cup (200ml) low-fat milk = 5	2 heaped tsp NESQUIK = 2			7
Berry smoothie	⅔ cup (150ml) skim milk = 3	¾ cup frozen berries = 3	100g diet vanilla yoghurt = 2	2 tsp wheat germ = 1	9
Regular shake	1 cup (250ml) milk = 8	1 tbsp chocolate syrup = 2			10
Skinny smoothie	⅔ cup (150ml) skim milk = 3	1 small banana = 4	100g diet vanilla yoghurt = 2	½ tbsp wheat germ = 1	10
Regular smoothie	¾ cup (200ml) regular milk = 6	1 small banana = 4	1 scoop vanilla ice cream = 5	2 tsp honey + ½ tbsp wheat germ = 3	18
Regular iced chocolate	¾ cup (200ml) regular milk = 6	2 scoops vanilla ice cream = 10	1 tbsp (20ml) chocolate syrup = 2	1 heaped tbsp whipped cream = 3	21
MILO milk	¾ cup (200ml) reduced fat milk = 5	3 tsp MILO (20g) = 4			9

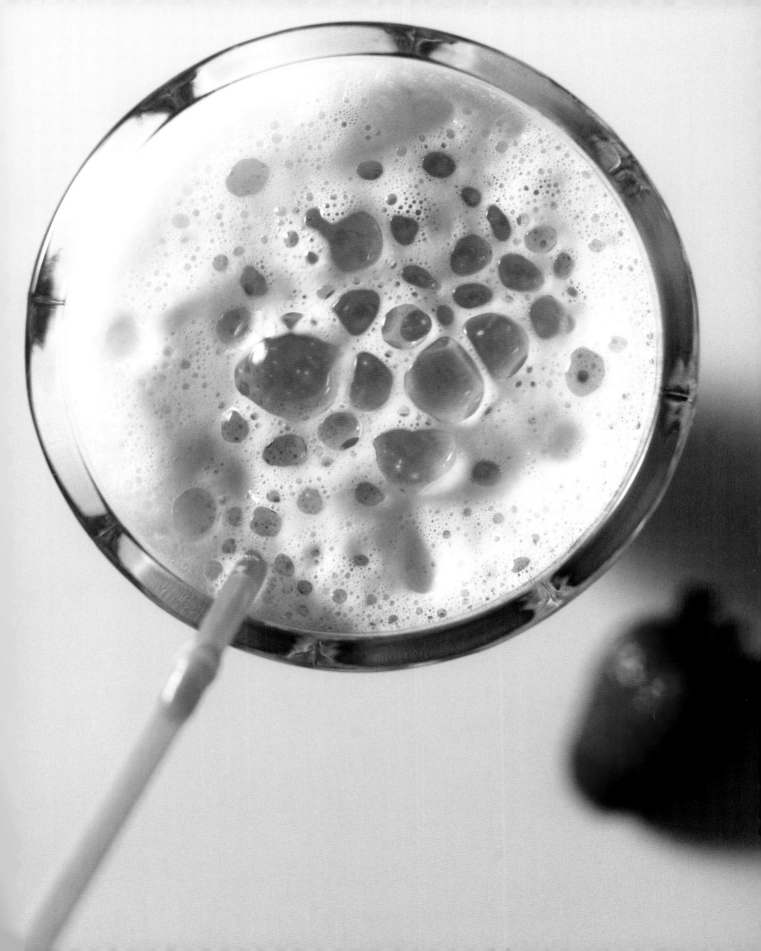

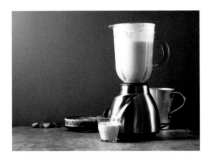

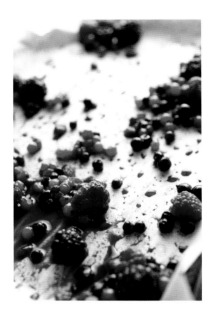

Our top five smoothie and juice combos for 10 counts or less

Any fruit smoothie (10 counts) 1 SERVE
¾ cup (200ml) skim milk
100g carton low-fat vanilla yoghurt
2 tsp wheat germ
1 medium banana OR ½ cup strawberries OR 1 large peach OR
   1 small peeled mango

1 Put all the ingredients in a blender, blend until frothy,
   then drink immediately.

Peach and mango thick shake (8 counts) 2 SERVES
1 cup (250ml) skim milk
1 scoop PETERS Light & Creamy Ice Cream
200g tub low-fat peach and mango yoghurt
½ cup sliced peaches in natural juice, drained.

1 Put all the ingredients in a blender, blend until frothy,
   then drink immediately.

Tropical fruit freeze (7 counts) 2 SERVES
1 cup (250ml) tropical fruit juice
200g carton low-fat mango yoghurt
1 large ripe banana
4 ice cubes (optional)

1 Put all the ingredients in a blender, blend until frothy,
   then drink immediately.

The kick-starter juice combo (6 counts) 1 SERVE
1 small carrot
1 small orange
3 celery sticks
1 small beetroot
1cm root ginger

1 Put all the ingredients in a juicer, juice and serve.

Refreshing juice combo (9 counts) 1 SERVE
300g watermelon
1 small punnet (250g) strawberries
1 apple or orange

1 Put all ingredients in a juicer, juice and serve.

Juice and cordials

Fruit juice

A large glass of fruit juice (650ml) is roughly equivalent to eating four to six pieces of whole fruit (depending on the fruit), provides around 8–16 counts and is consumed in minutes. Eating a piece of fruit, on the other hand, provides only 2–4 counts and can take up to 10 minutes to consume. The downside of a juice is that the fibre you would normally get from having a whole piece of fruit is absent, so you miss out on the natural 'full' sensation you would get if you were to eat the whole fruit. Although it may say 'no added sugar' on the label, fruit juice still contains natural sugars and provides around the same counts as soft drinks or cordials per serve. It does contain vitamins and minerals, though.

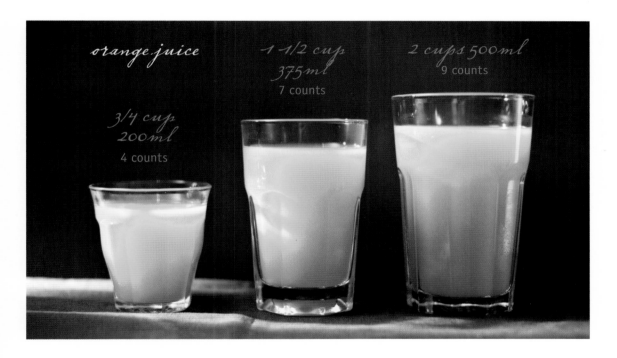

Vegetable juice

Vegetable juice also lacks the fibre you'd get from eating the vegetables themselves, but it is a lower count alternative to fruit juice. Watch out for store-bought vegetable juices, however, as they can contain added sodium (salt). Vegetable and fruit juice combos will have higher counts.

Soft drinks and cordials

Soft drinks and cordials contain a lot of added sugar and kilojoules (7 counts per 375ml) and virtually no other nutrients. Limit intake to special occasions or swap to low-calorie or diet alternatives if you drink these on a regular basis.

Energy drinks are as high in sugar as regular soft drinks while also containing high levels of caffeine per serve (higher than coffee and tea) and very little in the way of any extra nutrients.

Sports drinks are specially designed to help with rehydration, but they do contain a lot of counts, and unless you are a super athlete doing endurance events they are best avoided. As kids are more prone to dehydration, they can be useful to get kids to drink more fluids during extended activity such as sporting carnivals.

Alcohol

Alcohol is high in counts, having twice the number of kilojoules as either protein or carbohydrate per serve. It also causes the body to lose more water through the kidneys, so is dehydrating. In health terms, if you choose to drink alcohol, it's recommended we have no more than one standard drink a day. Plus we should aim to have at least two alcohol-free days a week.

When it comes to managing your weight, limit or avoid alcohol. Besides contributing excess counts, alcohol slows down your fat metabolism, encourages fat storage, can stimulate your appetite and weaken your resolve!

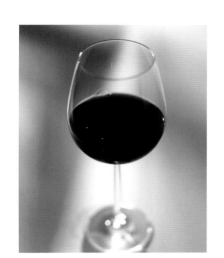

COCKTAIL AND DRINKS MATHS

Cosmopolitan = 7	60ml vodka = 6	+ 30ml cranberry juice = 1	+ dash lime juice = 0	+ ice = 0
Mojito = 10	60ml white rum = 7	+ 1 tbsp caster sugar = 3	+ 125ml soda water = 0	+ dash lime juice = 0
Whisky and dry = 5	30ml whisky = 3	+ 125ml ginger ale = 2	+ dash lime juice = 0	+ ice = 0
Bourbon and diet coke = 3	30ml bourbon = 3	+ 125ml diet coke = 0	+ ice = 0	
Shirley Temple = 4	15ml grenadine = 2	+ soda water = 0	+ 125ml ginger ale = 2	
Wine spritzer = 4	120ml white wine = 4	+ 200ml soda water = 0	+ slice lime = 0	
Shandy = 4	100ml full-strength beer = 2	+ 100ml lemonade = 2		

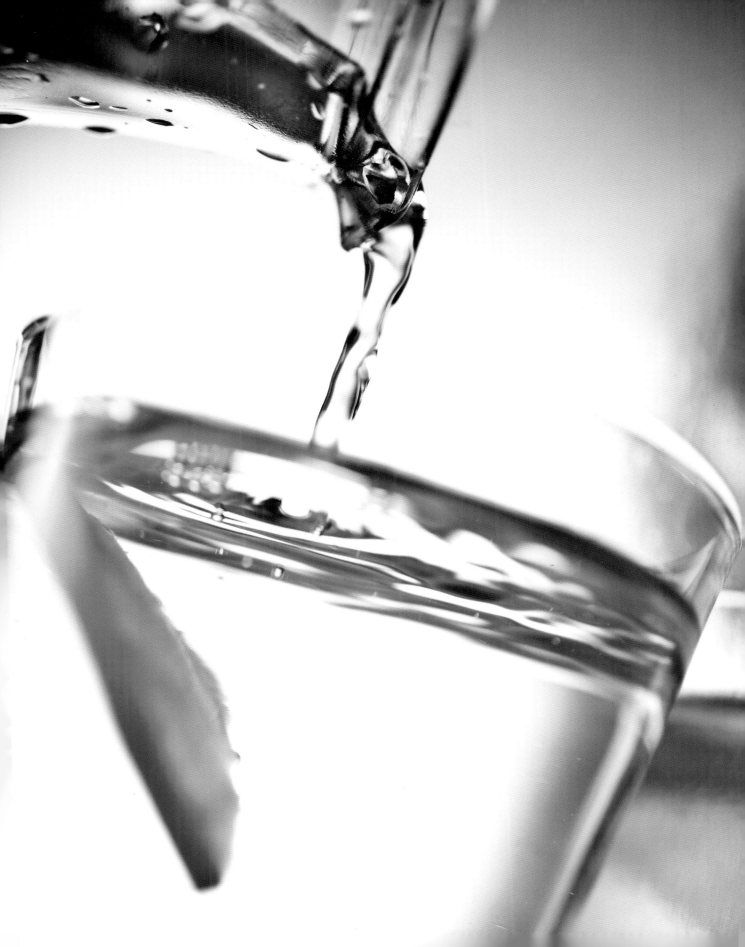

A–Z DRINKS COUNTER: HOW MANY COUNTS DOES YOUR FAVOURITE DRINK HAVE?

Fizzy drinks and mixers

Cinema 'extra large' 1 litre cup soft drink	21
Coca Cola, 375ml can	8
Coca Cola Buddy, 600ml	12
Deep Spring Mineral Water Lemon, 375ml	6
Ginger beer, 375ml	8
Mountain Dew, 250ml	6
7-Eleven Slurpee, Coca-Cola Classic, 500ml	7
Soda water, 375ml	0
Solo regular, 375ml	9
Tonic water, 375ml	6

Energy and vitamin drinks

Gatorade, 600ml	7
Glaceau Vitamin water, 500ml	5
Lucozade, 300ml	10
Mother energy drink, 500ml	11
PowerAde, 600ml	9
Red Bull, 250ml	6
V Energy Drink, 250ml	6

Fruit and vegetable drinks

Berri Multi-V, 400ml	7
Boost Juice Original Mango Magic Low-Fat Smoothie, 650ml	21
Boost Juice Original Wild Berry Juice, 650ml	13
Daily Juice Co. Classic Orange, 400ml	9
Just Juice Orange & Mango, 250ml	5
KFC Mango Smoothie Krusher, 380ml	19
Ribena, 250ml	5
V8 Tropical, 250ml	5
Velish Winter Vegetable Soup, 250g	6

Iced tea

Lipton Iced Green Tea, 500ml	7
NESTEA Lemon, 500ml	6

Milk and milk drinks

Big M Chocolate Milk, 600ml	20
Breaka Chocolate Flavoured Milk, 600ml	26
Dairy Farmers Rise Smoothie, 260ml	10
Dare Cappuccino iced coffee, 500ml	16
Dare Espresso, 500ml	20
Milk, regular tetrapak, 150ml	5
Moove Flavoured Milk Double Chocolate, 500ml	21
Moove Smooth Chocolate, 500ml	15
Oak flavoured milk, 500ml	20
Oak flavoured milk, 600ml	24
Sanitarium So Good Bliss Chocolate Soy Milk, 250ml	7
Sanitarium Up & Go, 350ml	14
Sustagen Mega Choc Ready to Drink, 250ml	14

Alcohol

Bacardi Breezer Lemon, 275ml	8
Bundaberg Rum & Cola, 375ml	12
Cougar Bourbon & Cola (5% alc), 375ml	11
Hahn Premium, 375ml	7
Hahn Premium Light, 375ml	5
Heineken, 330ml	6
Jim Beam & Cola Black Label, 375ml	11
Pure Blonde, 355ml	5
Smirnoff Ice Red (5% alc), 335ml	10
Standard glass wine (12% alc), 100ml	3
Strongbow Original Cider, 355ml	9
UDL Vodka, 375ml	11
VB full strength, 375ml	7

Coffee chains

Gloria Jeans Chai Tea, 300ml, regular milk	12
Gloria Jeans Hot Chocolate, 300ml, no cream	15
Gloria Jeans Regular Vanilla Honey Skim Chai Latte, 342ml, no whipped cream	9
Starbucks Caffe Latte Grande, 473ml, whole milk	13
Starbucks Caramel Macchiato, 473ml, whole milk	13
Starbucks Frappuccino Blended Strawberries & Cream Grande with whipped cream	21
Starbucks Grande Frappuccino, 473ml	11

Tips to manage alcohol when out:

- If you are thirsty, quench your thirst first with non-alcoholic drinks.
- Include non-alcoholic and low-calorie drinks, preferably water, between drinks.
- Watch out for the size of the glass. It is likely that the bigger the glass, the more you will serve yourself.
- When having mixed drinks, be careful what you mix it with.
- Choose low-alcohol beers, and if you drink wine try a spritzer (wine mixed with sparkling soda water).

PORTIONS HAVE TRIPLED—DRINKS HAVE BECOME MEALS

The size of the drinks we purchase has increased over the years. In the 1950s the standard soft drink container was 200ml, which increased to a 375ml can and, more recently, to a 600ml bottle. Head into a cinema and you are now offered the 1 litre cup! It has been proven that we will drink more if it is provided in a bigger container.

Did you know that soft drinks, juices, flavoured mineral waters, fruit-based drinks and sports drinks are the major source of sugar in our diet, and altogether provide about 30% of our added sugar intake?

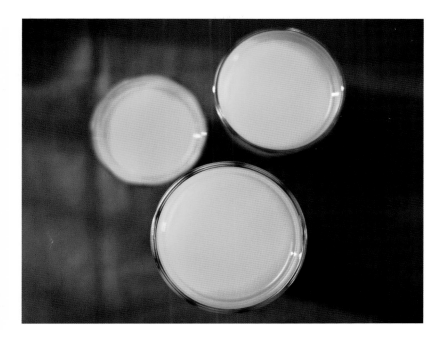

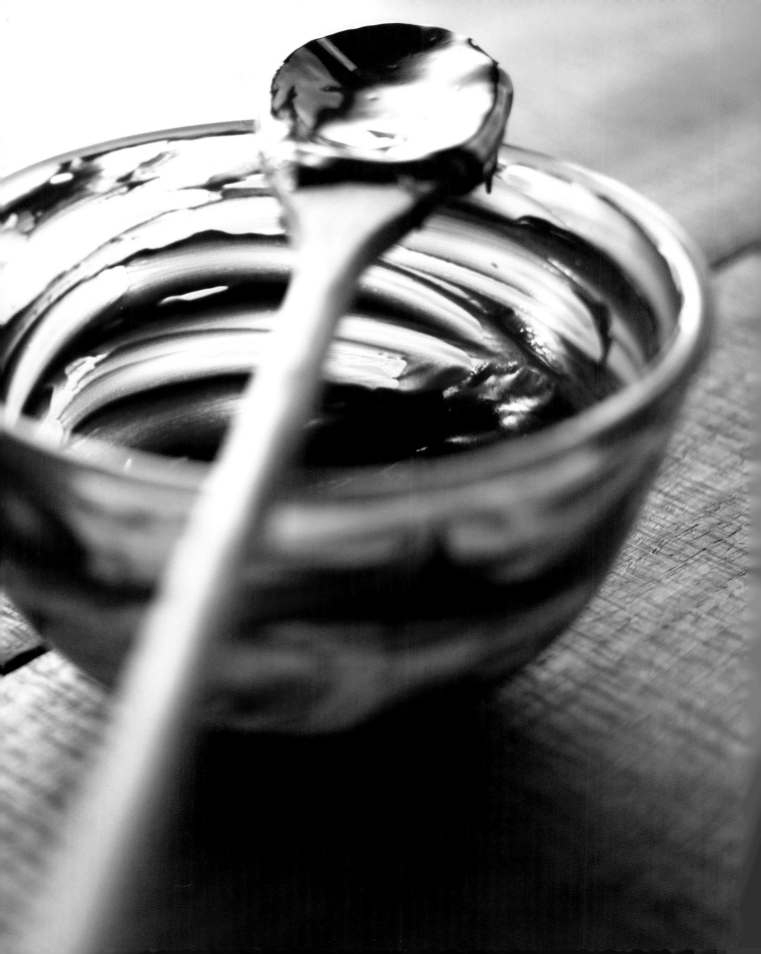

Both kids and grown-ups can occasionally enjoy delicious treats and desserts as part of a healthy, balanced diet. In fact, if you are active it's OK to enjoy a treat like some ice cream or a couple of squares of dark chocolate each day. Of course, treats don't always have to be food, but however you play it, treats are an important part of life.

Treats and desserts
for food lovers

Add fun and enjoyment to your day. A treat in your day can be an enjoyable detour in a healthy diet. It can boost both body and soul.

Celebrate special occasions. If you want to pull out all the stops and celebrate a special occasion, go for it and savour each mouthful.

Create memories. Food is so much more than what you put in your mouth. It is the squeals of delight as the birthday cake with candles glowing is proudly carried out from the kitchen to the resounding tones of Happy Birthday.

It's good to remember: Treats are optional extras and not everyone needs a treat each day. For those who do, 5 to 10 counts of treats can fit comfortably into most people's day, with bigger treats kept for special occasions.

Q&A

Q: Help, I crave chocolate. What can I do?

A: Sometimes cravings are just habits. We may feel like nibbling on a sweet biscuit or chocolate bar during our tea or coffee break simply because that's what we do every day—it's a bit like operating on autopilot. Here's a simple test. Wait at least 30 minutes before you eat the treat. Chances are you will have forgotten all about it before the time is up. At other times, we eat treats because they are there. One way to break the cycle is by not stocking them at home or at work.

When it comes to treat foods, it is better to enjoy a small portion occasionally than to try and ban it completely from your life. Making a food like chocolate taboo usually has the opposite effect—we crave it even more, eventually going overboard and binge eating a whole box. One strategy to take control of your cravings is to plan your treats. Building them into your week—whipping up a creamy dessert on Saturday night, or sharing a bar of chocolate on Sunday while watching a movie with friends—works for many people.

As for chocolate, think dark. Darker chocolate has a strong and rich flavour, which means you tend to crave less after the first mouthful. What's more, you'll get more of the good antioxidants! REALLY treat yourself and buy the best quality chocolate. Quality definitely beats quantity, so get the good stuff and appreciate it!

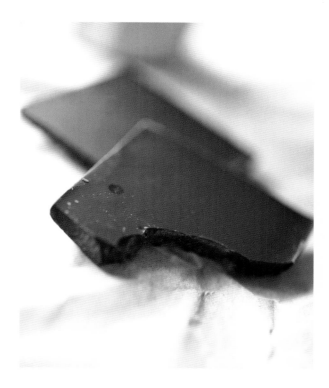

Fruit muffins and banana bread are better than cakes

Wrong! Fruit muffins and banana bread are still cakes! Most muffins and fruit cakes contain the same counts as chocolate cake and can cost you up to 27 counts depending on the portion size.

Yoghurt and frozen yoghurt are better than ice cream and gelato

Not always. Yoghurt and frozen yoghurt may be high in sugar and fat, so check the counts of your favourite brands (and calcium contents) and choose wisely.

It's a treat

Treats you eat (or drink)—chocolate, cake, brownies, desserts, sausage rolls, pies, hot chips, crisps, sweet biscuits, Danish pastries, croissants, doughnuts, beer, wine, spirits and fizzy drinks—are extras because they are generally high in fat and/or sugar and salt, and they usually come with double-figure counts. As we said in the snacks chapter, they are extras as they generally don't give us the essential nutrients our body needs.

However, you can enjoy occasional or regular treats by really savouring a small amount of something you love. Here are our tips to help you enjoy treats without blowing the count budget:

- ✓ The best place for treats is away from home, where there are no leftovers or other portions left in the bag or box to tempt you!
- ✓ Sharing is caring. Share a treat with friends or family. It's fun and means you won't eat the other half!
- ✓ Pick the portion-controlled options where you can—have a cupcake rather than cutting a slice of cake for yourself.
- ✓ Watch out for anything in pastry, or topped with a crumble or shortbread. These buttery options usually come with very high counts.

Myth buster

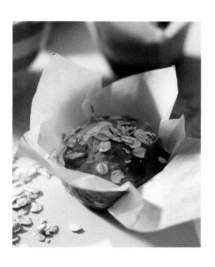

Neat treats

At home

- A 'fun pack' of KIT KAT (17g) = 4 counts, or SMARTIES (13g) = 3 counts. Individually wrapped means you can't go wrong with estimating what's a serve.
- Single-serve ice creams from ice cream multi-packs—a SKINNY COW Sundae Cup, for example, has 5 counts.
- A baby cupcake (or mini muffin). If you like to bake cupcakes, don't smother them in icing, simply dust with icing sugar. One regular-sized cupcake has about 7 counts.

Out and about

- In the mood for chocolate? Buy a truffle (yes, just one) at your favourite chocolate shop to take home or to enjoy with an espresso, cup of tea or skinny cappuccino or latte.
- Opt for the small sweet treats such as a macaroon (5 counts) to have with a coffee or tea instead of a slice of cake or a muffin.
- On hot days cool down with an icy treat like a FROSTY FRUITS or BILLABONG—they have 4 counts or less.

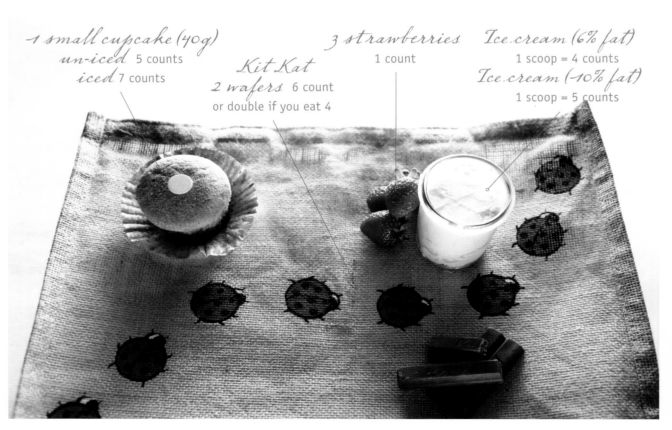

1 small cupcake (40g)
un-iced 5 counts
iced 7 counts

Kit Kat
2 wafers 6 count
or double if you eat 4

3 strawberries
1 count

Ice cream (6% fat)
1 scoop = 4 counts
Ice cream (~10% fat)
1 scoop = 5 counts

Better-for-you treats
- Choose an ice cream that's a source of calcium (check the label—not all are).
- Chocolate fondues are a great way of having a treat with your fruit! Cover one third of a large strawberry with dark chocolate and enjoy! You can also dip them in a flavoured yoghurt.
- Seafood can be a truly indulgent pleasure—oysters are rich in zinc, and a slice of smoked salmon has omega-3.
- And let's not forget dark chocolate and its antioxidants. Just two squares slowly savoured is amazingly satisfying.

What's in my ice cream?

Ice cream can be high in fat (10% fat) and also sugar. A regular (50g) scoop of vanilla ice cream will add about 5 counts. Some may be a source of calcium, but check the nutrition information panel to make sure. Check the ready-reckoner for the counts per scoop of your favourite brand.

COOL TREAT COUNTDOWN (1 SCOOP = 50G = 100ML)	
1 lemonade ICY POLE	2
1 scoop low-fat sorbet	3
1 scoop low-fat light and creamy ice cream	3
1 scoop gelato	3
1 single soft-serve frozen yoghurt	4
1 scoop regular frozen yoghurt	4
1 SKINNY COW English Toffee Stick	4
1 scoop regular vanilla ice cream	5
1 scoop milk-based sorbet	5
1 scoop super premium/rich ice cream	9
1 choc top regular ice cream	15
Cones add counts:	
Single cone (empty)	1
Large waffle cone (empty)	4

'DIS-COUNT' INDULGENCES

Treats don't need to be edible. Indulge your other senses—sight, sound, smell and touch—for the healthiest possible treats.

See

- Cuddle up on your couch or go out to watch a movie.
- Read a book or a magazine.
- Watch a play at the theatre.
- Go to an art gallery.
- Buy flowers for your home.
- Watch the sun rise or set while listening to your favourite music.

Listen

- Download a new music track to your iPod.
- Go to a concert!
- Get tickets for the opera.
- Phone or skype friends or family.
- Find something that makes you and your friends laugh—one of the best sounds of all.
- Get a bubbling water feature for your house or garden.

Smell

- Light some incense or scented candles.
- Use your favourite perfume mid-morning to give yourself a mood boost.
- Iron your sheets with linen spray for that 5 star hotel feeling.
- Have you bought those flowers yet?
- Aromatherapy lamps can do wonders!

Touch

- Take a hot bath with bath oil or salts. Don't forget music and candles!
- Treat yourself to a massage: scalp, hand or whole body.
- Have a pedicure, manicure, facial or other beauty TREATment from a professional or a caring friend.
- Book an appointment with your hairdresser.
- Wear your favourite silk shirt or cashmere jumper.
- Cuddle your dog or cat.
- Take off your shoes and take a walk on the beach or across the lawn.
- Start a carpentary project out in the back shed.

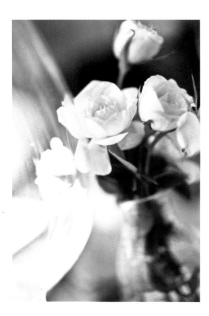

Count your treats

The cost of supersizing plain potato chips
20g packet = 6 counts
50g packet = 12 counts
100g packet = 24 counts
200g packet = 48 counts

I'll have cream with that
1 tbsp double cream = 4 counts
1 tbsp thickened cream = 3 counts
1 tbsp lite cream = 2 counts
1 tbsp aerosol can of cream = 3 counts

Quick-fix lolly treats

Here's what you get for 5 counts of your favourite lollies

LOLLY	NUMBER OF PIECES
Jelly beans	12 jelly beans
SNAKES ALIVE	2 snakes
Party mix	6 pieces
ALLEN'S reduced sugar snakes	5 snakes
Red frogs	7 small or 4 big
Lollipops	2 lollipops
KOOL Fruits	7 pieces
LIFE SAVERS (5 flavour)	12 pieces
Jubes	5 pieces
Liquorice allsorts	5 pieces (35g)
Boiled lollies	6 small (5g a piece)
Marshmallows	6 small (5g a piece)

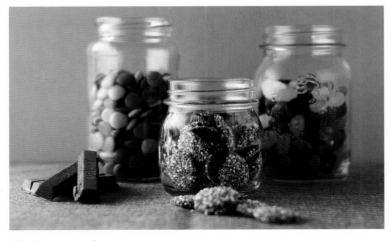

The key to good treats is portion size

Food	Counts
1 fortune cookie	2
1 lemonade ice block	2
½ cup of jelly	4
1 slice of garlic bread	4
1 shortbread biscuit	4
1 small wedge (30g) of camembert	4
1 party-size sausage roll	6
1 plain scone	5
1 chocolate Tim Tam	5
1 macaroon biscuit	5
1 party-size meat pie	5
3 sticks of liquorice	6
1 slice (40g) sponge swiss roll	6
1 McDonalds ice cream and cone	7
1 small cupcake with icing	7
1 small friand	8
1 piece of baklava (50g)	10
1 medium muffin	10
1 chocolate brownie	11
1 finger bun with icing	12
1 cinnamon doughnut	12
1 medium piece of vanilla slice	13
1 slice of pavlova with cream and fruit	13
6 chicken nuggets	14
1 small cup (150g) of hot potato chips	14
1 slice of lemon meringue pie	15
1 slice of chocolate bavarian	15
1 choc top ice cream	15
1 McDonalds regular Hot Fudge Sundae	16
1 individual custard tart	17
1 individual apple pie, 150g	17
1 large sausage roll	18
1 spring roll	19
1 slice of caramel slice	19
1 slice of chocolate mud cake with icing	21
1 regular meat pie	22
1 slice of pecan pie	22
1 large chocolate eclair	23
1 scone with jam and cream	23
1 apple and custard scroll	23
1 large container of cinema popcorn	26

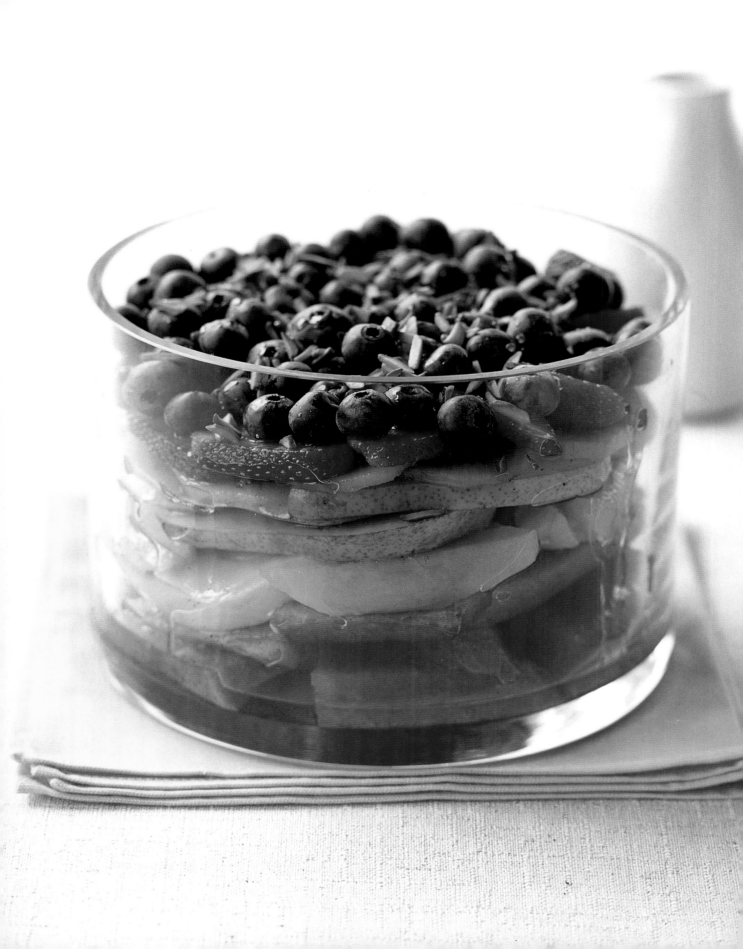

Treats and dessert recipes

Layered summer fruits

800g watermelon, peeled and sliced

2 mangoes, sliced

2 pears, sliced

3 kiwi fruit, peeled and sliced

250g strawberries, hulled and sliced

150g fresh or frozen blueberries

½ cup freshly squeezed orange juice (optional)

Lemon pistachio syrup

1 vanilla bean, split and scraped, or 1 teaspoon vanilla essence

½ cup caster sugar

2 tsp lemon zest

1 tsp rosewater essence

50g pistachio kernels, roughly chopped

1 Layer fruits in a large serving bowl.
2 Place the vanilla bean (or vanilla essence), sugar, lemon zest, rosewater essence and 1 ½ cups of water in a saucepan and bring to the boil. Reduce heat and simmer for 15 minutes or until slightly thickened. Allow to cool then strain.
3 Pour the syrup over the fruits. Sprinkle with pistachios and garnish with yogurt if desired.
4 Alternatively, to save counts, replace the syrup with ½ cup freshly squeezed orange juice.

Fruit platters—there's nothing more indulgent or inviting than seasonal fruits beautifully presented.

PREP: 25 mins
MAKES: 6
COUNTS PER SERVE: 13 (with syrup)
COUNTS PER SERVE: 7 (with orange juice and without the syrup)

French crepes with berries

PREP: 15 mins
COOK: 15 mins
SERVES: 6
COUNTS PER SERVE: 11
1 SCOOP LOW-FAT ICE CREAM =
    3 counts

Berry sauce

½ punnet blueberries

½ punnet strawberries, hulled and halved

¼ cup caster sugar

1 tsp vanilla essence

1 cup water

2 tsp cornflour

French crepes

½ cup plain flour

1 tbsp caster sugar

20g butter or margarine, melted

1 tsp grated lemon rind, optional

2 eggs

¾ cup CARNATION Light & Creamy Evaporated Milk

oil spray

Berry sauce

1 Place the berries, sugar, vanilla and water in a saucepan, and bring to the boil. Reduce the heat to low and cook for 3 minutes, or until the sugar dissolves.

2 Dissolve the cornflour in 1 tablespoon of water to make a paste. Stir into the berry sauce and simmer, stirring constantly, for 2 minutes or until the sauce thickens, then cover and remove from the heat.

French crepes

1 Sift the flour into a bowl and stir in the sugar. Combine the butter, lemon rind, eggs and evaporated milk in a jug. Whisk into the flour and stir until smooth.

2 Lightly spray a non-stick frying pan with oil, and place over medium heat. Pour in ¼ cup of the batter and tilt the pan so the mixture makes a thin circle. Cook for 2 minutes, then flip the crepe and cook on the other side until golden. Remove the crepe from the pan and transfer to a low oven to keep warm while you cook the remaining crepes.

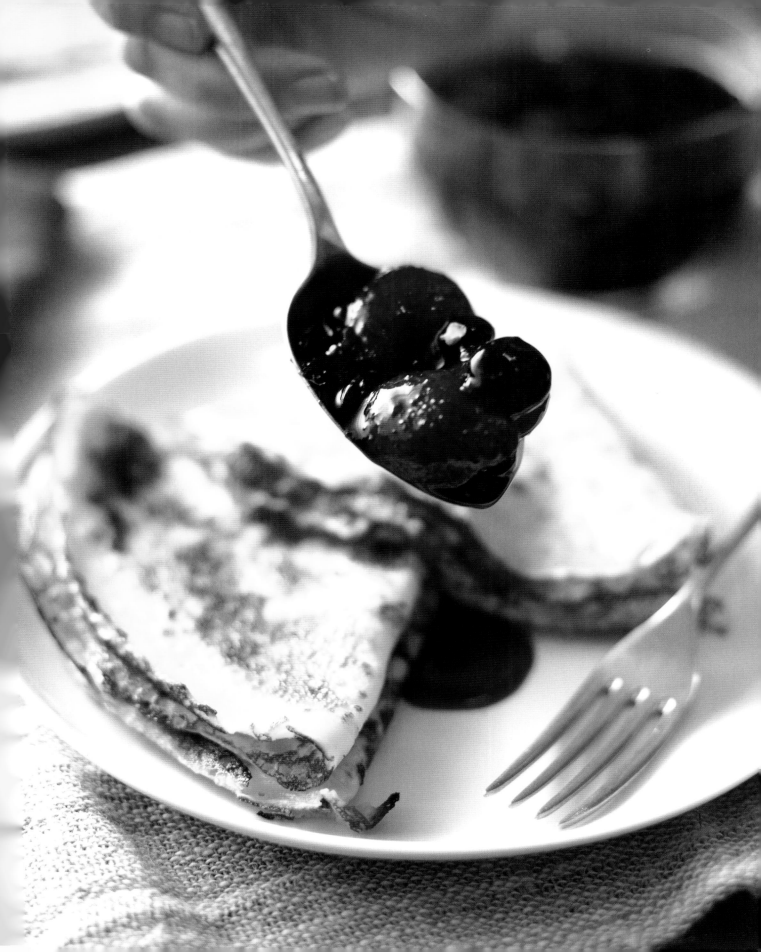

Dairy-free custard tart

You can use soy cooking milk to make this tart dairy free, but it's just as delicious with regular evaporated milk if you prefer.

PREP: 45 mins
COOK: 60 mins (plus cooling time)
SERVES: 10
COUNTS PER SERVE: 12

Pastry

2 cups plain flour

¼ cup caster sugar

60g dairy-free spread

2 egg yolks

3 tbsp water

Custard filling

375ml CARNATION Soy Creamy Cooking Milk

3 eggs, lightly beaten

1 tsp vanilla extract

¼ cup caster sugar

1 tsp cornflour

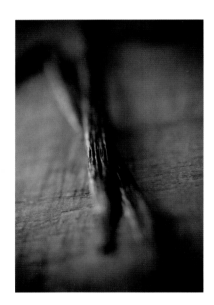

1 To make the pastry, combine the flour, sugar and dairy-free spread in a food processor, and process until the mixture resembles fine breadcrumbs. Add the egg yolks and water, and process until the dough just starts to come together. Turn the dough onto a lightly floured surface. Knead for 10 minutes until almost smooth. Cover and refrigerate for 30 minutes.

2 Preheat the oven to 200°C (180°C fan-forced). Place the dough between two sheets of baking paper and roll out to a 28cm disc. Line a round 23cm tart tin with pastry and trim off the excess. Lightly prick the base with a fork, cover the pastry with baking paper and fill with dried beans or uncooked rice. Bake for 15 minutes, then carefully remove the paper and beans/rice from the pastry case and bake for a further 10 minutes. Remove the pastry case from the oven and cool. Reduce the oven temperature to 160°C (140°C fan-forced).

3 To make the custard filling, place the soy cooking milk in a saucepan to simmer. Whisk together the eggs, vanilla, sugar and cornflour, and pour over the warmed milk. Strain the liquid into the tart shell. Bake in the oven for 30 minutes or until firm, then cover and refrigerate overnight.

4 Serve with fresh berries.

Chocolate ice Cream

375ml can CARNATION Creamy Evaporated Milk, chilled overnight
½ cup chocolate topping
1 tsp vanilla essence
100g PLAISTOWE Dark Cooking Chocolate, grated

1 Using an electric mixer, beat the evaporated milk until thick and frothy. Add the chocolate topping, vanilla and dark cooking chocolate, then beat until well combined.
2 Pour the mixture into a deep 1.5 litre (6 cup) container and freeze overnight, or until firm. Alternatively, pour the whipped mixture into an ice cream maker and churn according to the manufacturer's instructions.

Ice cream is a popular treat for many of us at the end of the day and is especially good with some fresh or canned fruit. When there's time, it's fun and easy to make your own—especially if you have an ice cream maker.

PREP: 5 mins (plus refrigeration
   and freezing time)
MAKES: 1.5 litres (6 cups)
SERVES: 15 scoops
COUNTS PER SCOOP: 4

Peach and raspberry ice cream

375ml CARNATION Creamy Evaporated Milk, chilled overnight
410g can peach slices, drained and pureed
½ cup frozen raspberries
¼ cup sugar

1 Using an electric mixer, beat the evaporated milk until thick and frothy. Add the peach puree, raspberries and sugar, and beat until well combined.
2 Pour the mixture into a deep 1.5 litre (6 cup) container and freeze overnight, or until firm. Alternatively, pour the whipped mixture into an ice cream maker and churn according to the manufacturer's instructions.

PREP: 5 mins (plus refrigeration
   and freezing time)
MAKES: 1.5 litres (6 cups)
SERVES: 15 scoops
COUNTS PER SCOOP: 3

PREP: 5 mins (plus refrigeration and freezing time)
MAKES: 1.5 litres (6 cups)
SERVES: 15 scoops
COUNTS PER SCOOP: 6

Cheesecakes can be very rich—a virtual calorie bomb. But this new take on an old favourite uses light cream cheese and light evaporated milk to give you plenty of calcium for your counts.

PREP: 20 mins
SETTING TIME: 3 hours
SERVES: 12
COUNTS PER SERVE: 12

Apricot ice cream

375ml CARNATION Creamy Evaporated Milk, chilled overnight

410g apricot halves, drained and pureed

300ml thickened cream

½ cup sugar

1 Using an electric mixer, beat the evaporated milk until thick and frothy. Fold in the apricot puree, cream and sugar until combined.
2 Pour the mixture into a deep 1.5 litre (6 cup) container and freeze overnight, or until firm. Alternatively, pour the whipped mixture into an ice cream maker and churn according to the manufacturer's instructions.

Light berry cheesecake

125g plain sweet biscuits, crushed

60g margarine, melted

375g light cream cheese

½ cup sugar

375ml CARNATION Light & Creamy Evaporated Milk

1 tsp vanilla essence

3 tsp gelatine

¼ cup hot water

300g mixed berries

1 Combine the biscuit crumbs and margarine, and mix well. Press the biscuit mix into the base of a 22cm springform tin and refrigerate until firm.
2 Beat the cream cheese and sugar until smooth. Gradually beat in the evaporated milk and vanilla essence.
3 In a separate bowl, dissolve the gelatine in hot water, then cool and beat into the cheesecake mixture. Pour the mixture over the biscuit base and refrigerate until set. Decorate with berries.

Coconut crème caramel

1 cup caster sugar

1 cup water

375ml CARNATION Light & Creamy Coconut Flavoured Milk

2 eggs

2 egg whites

1 Preheat the oven to 200°C (180°C fan-forced).
2 Place ¾ cup caster sugar and ½ cup of water in a saucepan, and boil until the colour turns to caramel, taking care not to burn. Pour into six ¾-cup capacity ovenproof moulds and set aside.
3 Whisk the coconut-flavoured milk, eggs, egg whites and the remaining sugar and water in a bowl, then strain into a jug and pour evenly into the moulds.
4 Place the ovenproof moulds into a baking dish and add boiling water to reach halfway up the sides of the moulds. Bake for 20 minutes or until just set, then refrigerate for 2 hours.
5 Turn out on serving dishes to serve.

By substituting coconut-flavoured evaporated milk (2% fat) for regular coconut milk (25% fat), you can save counts and add calcium to this popular treat.

PREP: 15 mins
COOK: 20 mins
SERVES: 6
COUNTS PER SERVE: 11

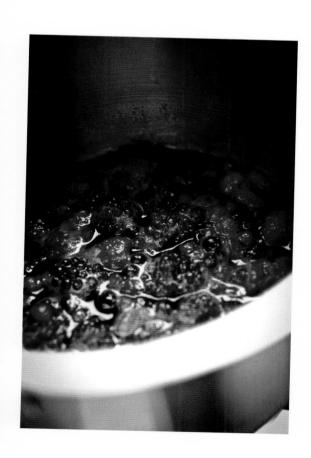

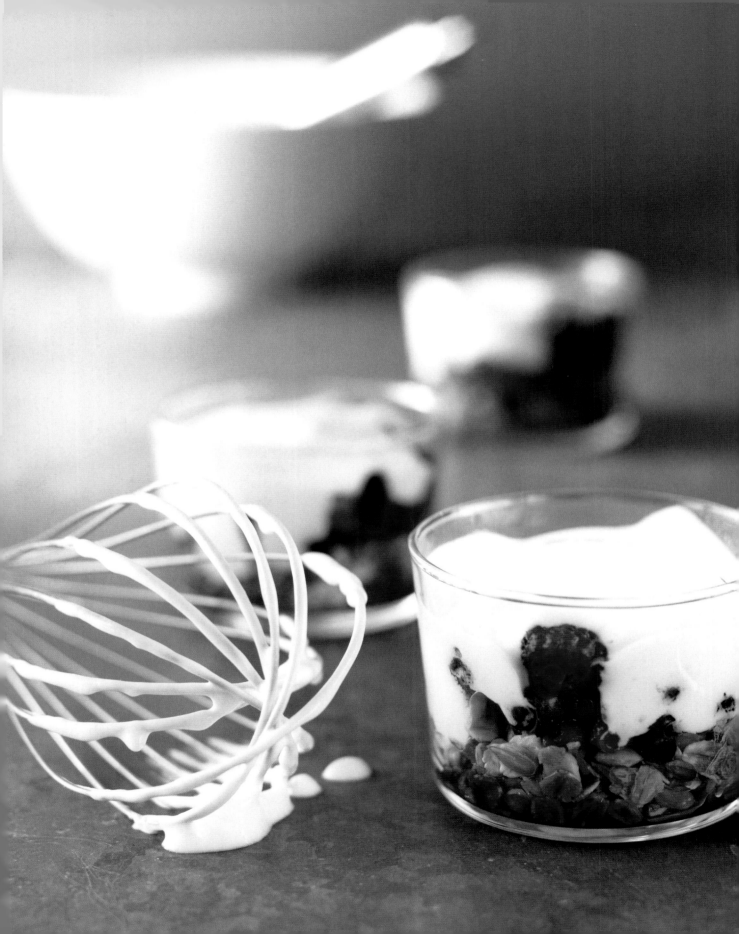

Whipped yoghurt berry crunch

1 cup UNCLE TOBYS Traditional Oats

¼ cup sunflower seeds

¼ cup pepitas (pumpkin seeds)

¼ cup shredded coconut

¼ cup flaked almonds

1 tbsp honey

2 cups frozen mixed berries, defrosted

800g diet vanilla yoghurt

There's an amazing range of tastes and textures in this easy and nourishing dessert. Just halve quantities to serve four.

PREP: 10 mins
COOK: 15 mins
SERVES: 8
COUNTS PER SERVE: 10

1 Preheat the oven to 160°C (140°C fan-forced).
2 Place the oats, sunflower seeds, pepitas, coconut and almonds on a tray, and roast for 10 minutes. Remove from the oven, drizzle with honey and roast for a further 5 minutes.
3 Meanwhile, pour the yoghurt into a bowl and whisk until light and fluffy. Then, in eight glasses, alternately layer the oat mixture, berries and yoghurt. Chill, or eat immediately.

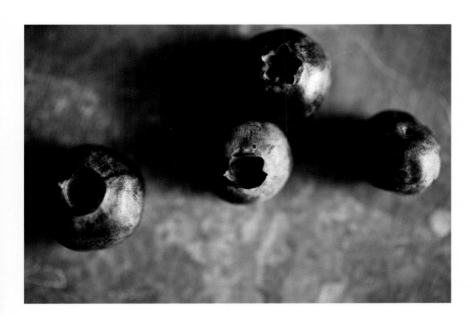

If you are a chocolate lover, switching to dark chocolate delivers a healthy dose of antioxidants. Making this delicious treat in individual moulds helps to keep those extra counts under control and means everyone gets their share.

PREP: 10 mins
SETTING TIME: 3 hours
SERVES: 4
COUNTS PER SERVE: 10

Four-ingredient chocolate mousse

100g 70% dark chocolate, chopped

2 tbsp water

10g unsalted butter

3 eggs, separated

1 In a small saucepan, bring a small quantity of water to the boil, place a heatproof bowl firmly on top of the saucepan, add the chocolate, water and butter, and stir until melted. Remove the bowl from the saucepan. Add the egg yolks to the chocolate mixture one at a time, stirring constantly.

2 In an electric mixer, whisk the egg whites until stiff peaks form. Gently fold the egg whites into the chocolate mixture. Spoon the mixture into four ¾-cup capacity moulds. Refrigerate for 3 hours, or until set.

TIP: HOW TO MELT CHOCOLATE

- Microwave method: Microwave chocolate in a microwave-proof dish, uncovered, on MEDIUM (50%) for 1 minute. Remove from the microwave, stir and repeat the process in 30 second intervals until the chocolate is melted.

- Stove top method: In a small saucepan, bring a small quantity of water to the boil, remove from the heat and place a heatproof bowl firmly on top of the pan. Place the chocolate in the heatproof bowl and stir until melted, allowing 4–6 minutes.

Use the melted chocolate in recipes as directed, or for dipping berries and fruit for a tasty treat at the end of dinner.

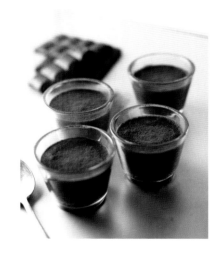

Tiramisu cake

1 tbsp gelatine

1½ cups low-fat ricotta

¼ cup skim milk

¼ cup caster sugar

2 tbsp instant coffee

⅓ cup boiling water

⅓ cup skim milk

½ cup coffee liqueur

250g savoiardi (ladyfinger) biscuits

1 Grease and line the base and sides of a 20cm round cake tin. Dissolve the gelatine in 1 tablespoon of boiling water, then leave to cool. Using an electric mixer, whisk the ricotta, milk (¼ cup), sugar and gelatine until smooth.

2 In a large bowl dissolve the instant coffee, boiling water, milk (⅓ cup) and liqueur. Soak the savoiardi biscuits in the coffee mixture and line the base of the cake tin with them. Carefully smooth half the ricotta mixture over the biscuits and repeat the process.

3 Refrigerate for 3 hours, or until set. Decorate with chocolate curls if desired.

This cake is ideal for special occasions, when entertaining or when you want to serve something different at a family get-together. Because it's made with low-fat ricotta and skim milk, it almost counts as a healthy indulgence!

PREP: 20 mins
SETTING TIME: 3 hours
SERVES: 8
COUNTS PER SERVE: 12

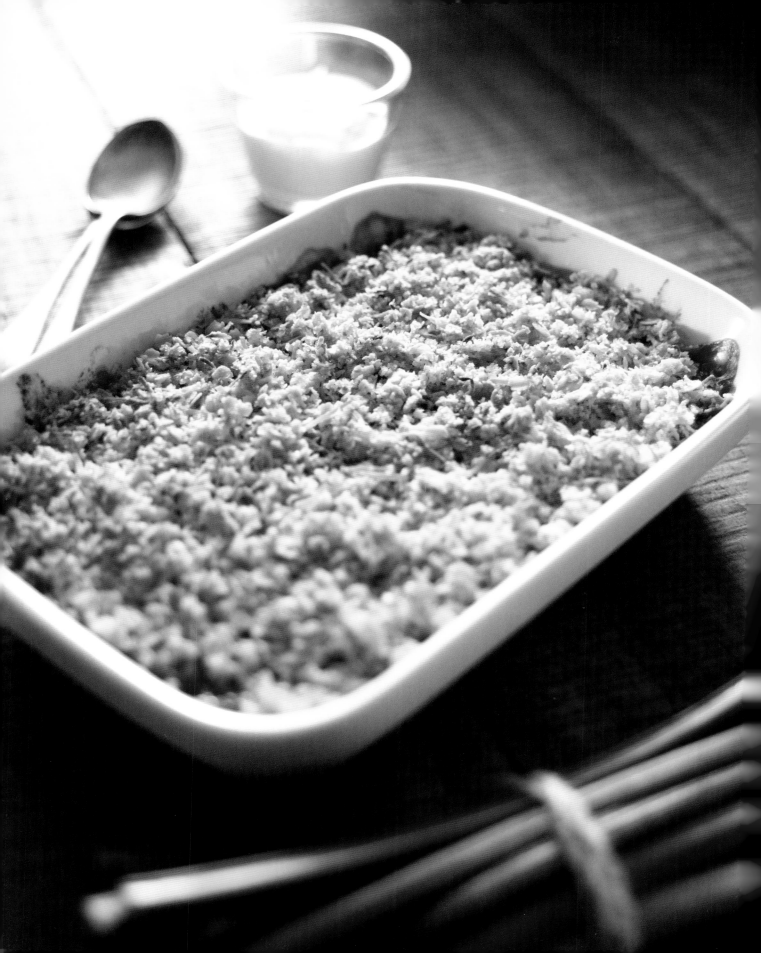

Pear and rhubarb crumble

1 bunch rhubarb, trimmed and cut into 5cm lengths

2 pears, cored, peeled and sliced

2 tbsp brown sugar

juice of half a lemon

1 tbsp water

1 cup UNCLE TOBYS Traditional Oats

⅓ cup shredded coconut

40g dairy-free spread

⅓ cup brown sugar, extra

1 Preheat the oven to 180°C (160°C fan-forced). Lightly grease a 6-cup capacity baking dish.

2 Combine the rhubarb, pear, sugar, juice and water in a medium saucepan. Cook the mixture, covered, for 5 minutes or until softened. Drain the fruit mixture and discard the liquid. Spoon the fruit into the prepared dish.

3 Place the oats, coconut, dairy-free spread and extra brown sugar in a medium-size bowl. Using fingertips, rub in the dairy-free spread until the mixture is crumbly. Sprinkle the dry mix over the fruit in the baking dish and bake in the oven for 15 minutes, or until golden.

This family favourite combines a crisp and crunchy topping with a fruity filling, and made our way it delivers a delicious dairy-free twist for non-dairy eaters. Serve with vanilla soy yoghurt if desired.

PREP: 10 mins
COOK: 20 mins
SERVES: 6
COUNTS PER SERVE: 10

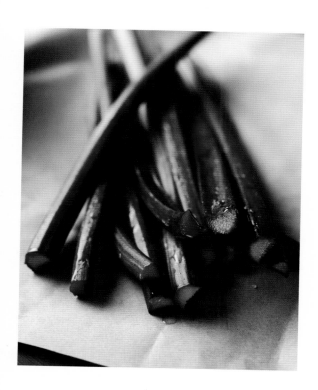

*Enjoy one of these treats
at home, or make them
for a picnic treat*

Chocolate chip and peanut butter cookies

PREP: 20 mins
COOK: 12 mins
MAKES: 24
COUNTS PER COOKIE: 8

125g butter, softened

⅓ cup peanut butter

1 cup brown sugar

1 egg

¼ cup baking cocoa

½ cup plain flour

¾ cup self-raising flour

250g NESTLÉ CHOC BITS, dark

1 Preheat the oven to 180°C (160°C fan-forced). Line two oven trays with baking paper.

2 Cream the butter, peanut butter and sugar together. Beat in the egg, stir in the cocoa and flours, then add half of the choc bits.

3 Roll heaped teaspoonfuls of the mixture into balls. Place the balls on the trays and press with a fork, then gently press the remaining choc bits on the tops.

4 Bake for 12 minutes until golden. Stand for 5 minutes before transferring to a wire rack to cool.

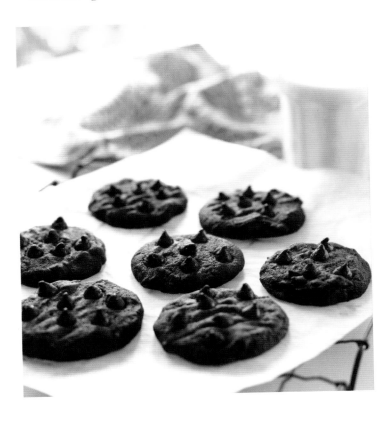

Mini gingerbread men

125g butter, cut into cubes

½ cup caster sugar

½ tsp ground ginger

2½ tsp ground cinnamon

¼ cup sweetened condensed milk

1 egg

2½ cups plain flour

1 tsp baking powder

Icing

2 tbsp sweetened condensed milk

¾ cup icing sugar

1 tbsp water

Decoration

100g SMARTIES

¼ cup NESTLÉ CHOC BITS, dark

silver cachous

March these mini iced gingerbread men into the hearts of those little people in your family. Teaching our children how to handle treat foods is giving them a gift that will stand them in good stead throughout their lives.

PREP: 20 mins
COOK: 12 mins
MAKES: 40
COUNTS PER MINI GINGERBREAD MAN: 5

1 Preheat the oven to 180°C (160°C fan-forced). Line two oven trays with baking paper.
2 Beat the butter and sugar together until light and creamy. Add the spices, condensed milk and egg, and mix well. Sift the flour and baking powder, and stir into the mixture. Mix until the dough forms a ball. Wrap the dough ball in plastic wrap and refrigerate for 10–15 minutes.
3 Cut the dough in half and roll out between sheets of baking paper to 5mm thick. Cut out gingerbread men (or other shapes) using a cutter. Repeat with the remaining dough. Place the biscuits on oven trays and bake in batches for 12–15 minutes, until golden. Cool for 5 minutes on the tray before transferring to a wire rack.

Icing

1 Mix together the condensed milk, icing sugar and water. Spread over the cold biscuits.
2 Decorate the biscuits using SMARTIES for buttons, choc bits for the mouth and silver cachous for eyes.

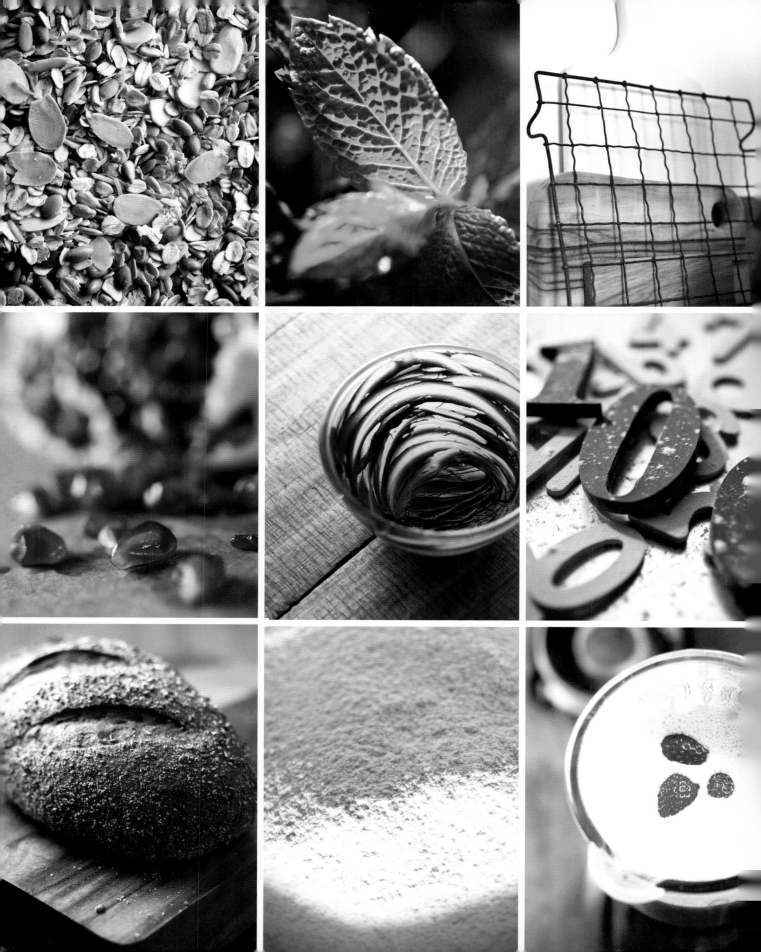

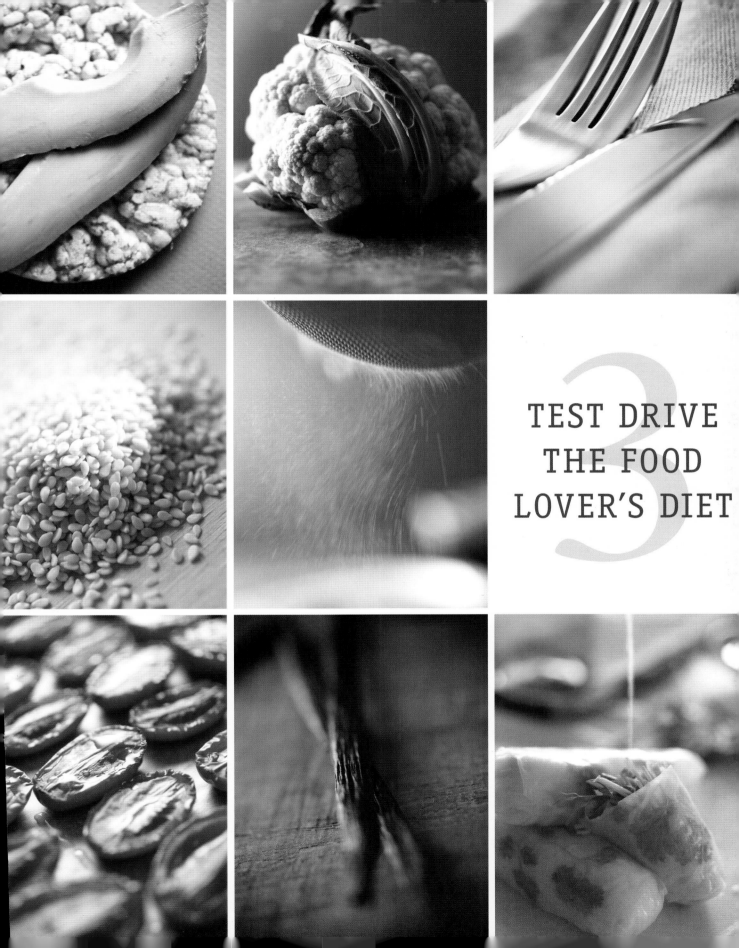

3

TEST DRIVE THE FOOD LOVER'S DIET

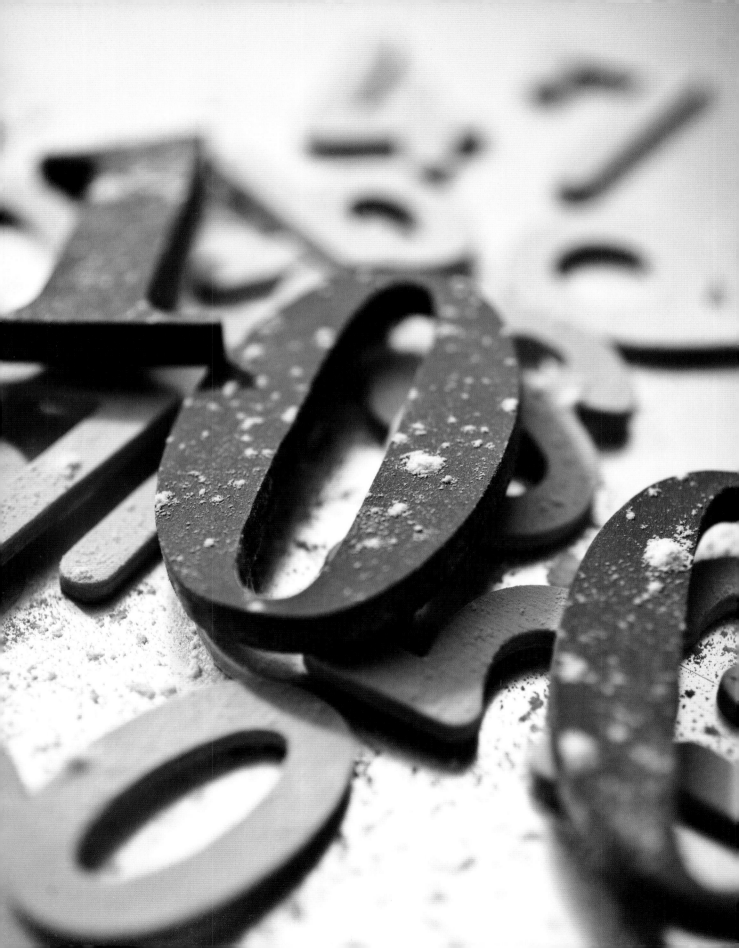

More and more we are realising that achieving a happy weight is not only about the food we eat. It's about how and why we eat. Often our food habits can reflect a chaos in other areas of our life. Work and family commitments, or simply being busy, stressed or disorganised can all affect the way we eat and can undermine our health. We eat when we are emotional, when we want a break, when we want to socialise or want to procrastinate! Basically, we often eat for many reasons beyond hunger, and these are the food habits that are worth changing.

Test drive
The Food Lover's Diet

It's good to remember: Quite simply, if you want life to be different you have to do things differently.

Succeeding to plan is planning to succeed. First things first. As silly as it sounds, to change you must want to change. It's not enough that others, like friends or family, want you to change.

You and you alone have to decide you will invest the time and effort in improving and supporting yourself. Because, until you are ready to change, you will do all in your (unconscious) power to sabotage yourself so you can stay safely, (un)happily, exactly where you are.

Remember, you will only change when you are mentally, emotionally and physically ready to.

Are you ready to change?

Change happens in stages. It will help you be successful in making changes if you check first to see if you're really ready to commit to change. Circle the statement below in the left-hand column that you think most applies to you. Then read across.

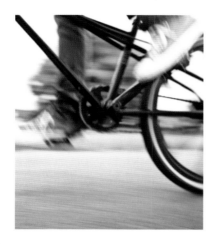

IS THIS YOU?	WHAT TO DO ...
Stage 1. 'I'm not thinking about change. I don't have plans to do anything differently in the near future.'	If this is you, write down all the pros and cons of changing or not changing. By listing the costs of staying the same versus the benefits of change, it may help you go on to Stage 2.
Stage 2. 'I'm thinking about the need to change but have no definite plans yet.'	Try brainstorming a list of barriers that may be stopping you from changing. Come up with some possible solutions or resources that would help take you to Stage 3.
Stage 3. 'I am preparing to change. I have started collecting ideas and information, I'm looking at options and I'm making plans to change.'	Write out a goal you would like to achieve (see our template on the next page) and identify an ACTION PLAN to go to Stage 4.
Stage 4. 'I'm putting my plan into action and have started doing some things differently.'	Great. Keep up the good work. You are well on the way to achieving your goal long term.
Stage 5. 'I'm doing these new behaviours regularly and have been maintaining my new habits.'	Congratulations! When you have been doing this for more than six months it is becoming a new way of life.

Remember, when it comes to maintaining good habits, success is as much about good problem-solving as it is about motivation. Invariably life throws you a curved ball, problems arise, you make a mistake and the good food or exercise habits fall to the wayside for a while. If this happens, you just need to be flexible and patient while you find different ways or new skills to keep achieving the same outcome. It's *not* about thinking you have failed or fallen off the bandwagon—it's simply about needing a new solution to meet new circumstances. When that happens, go back to stage 2 or 3 and devise a new plan, knowing you have done it before and can do it again!

Now, after those tips you should be in the right frame of mind to get started!

Setting a goal

No journey ever starts without first knowing where you want to go. What is it you want to achieve? Some may want to stay the same weight but get fitter, or stop their weight from seesawing up and down, while others might want to lose a few kilograms before the holidays.

Really, we all know what to do. The hard part is taking the time to be clear about how we are going to do it. What's the aim? What's the plan? And then let's be sure we get around to doing it! Taking the time to set SMART goals is a step towards success.

A goal needs to be specific. You need to state clearly: why, how, what, when and where you will undertake to do what you plan to do. If you have a vague goal, without any clear idea of how you will achieve it, it is less likely you will succeed.

Set SMART goals:

S - Be **s**pecific
M - **M**easure your progress
A - Be **a**ction oriented
R - Be **r**ealistic
T - Set a **t**imeframe

MY ACTION PLAN TO ACHIEVE MY GOAL

What I will do:

How I will do it:

When and where I will do it:

Why I want to do it:

EXAMPLE OF ACTION PLAN TO ACHIEVE MY GOAL

What I will do:	I will count everything I eat and drink for three days.
How I will do it:	I will buy a special notebook that fits into my bag and make sure I have a pencil or pen.
When and where I will do it:	I will carry it with me all the time for the three days and record everything I eat or drink, and in the evening I will set aside 30 minutes to work out the counts and tally up the day's total.
Why I want to do it:	I want to fit into my favourite jeans.

Regular monitoring helps you check your progress. Try setting up a grid like the one below.

Tracking my PROGRESS

DAY AND DATE	ACHIEVED (YES ☑ OR NO ☒)	REFLECTIONS OR COMMENTS
Day 1:	☐	
Day 2:	☐	
Day 3:	☐	

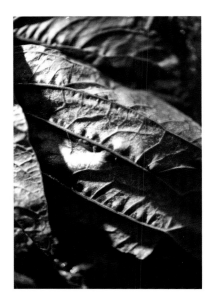

You now have some insight into your goals, you have the tools to achieve those goals, and all that's left is to just do it! Starting is often the hardest step of all—it is so much easier to just keep thinking about it. Physically picking up different foods in the supermarket, buying them, trying them, taking the time to learn how to prepare them, tasting them, then mentally preparing for the children whining when you put something different down in front of them, can seem daunting.

Change is often uncomfortable at first. New ways of eating and living can feel strange. For two weeks you may find you need to try a little harder to keep those new changes 'top of mind', then for the next six weeks it gets easier, and after six months it is almost a way of life and you may even become a zealot, unable to believe life was ever any other way!

We have written some menu plans on pages 217–20 to help you get started. Feel the benefits, maintain your focus and support your choices. Just start!

We have tried to make a simple template of options that include typical and popular meals—a framework of four choices for each meal with a suggested number of counts. So you can mix and match, be flexible and do and choose whatever suits you in that moment. Some of the meals use recipes from this book where the counts per serving are already calculated for you, whereas others are simple dishes you can whip up with what's on hand.

My mix-and-match menu plan

You can add up your counts as you go through the day. Alternatively you can create a menu plan by allocating your counts by meals as in the example below.

On pages 25–27 you will have worked out how many counts are right for you. Match that number to the table below. In the meal plans we have included snacks, and even a treat if you wish. If you prefer not to include these, just carry the counts over to another part of the day, making the meals bigger at the time of day that suits your counts total, your schedule, activity and hunger!

COUNTS PER MEAL	60 COUNTS	75 COUNTS	100 COUNTS	110 COUNTS
Breakfast	10	15	20	25
Lunch	15	20	25	25
Dinner	20	25	30	35
Snacks	10*	10*	15*	15*
Treats	5	5	10	10

*e.g. 10=2x5, 15=3x5

On days where you may be going out for lunch with friends or celebrating over dinner with family, you can choose to have more counts at that meal, then borrow some counts from an earlier meal or later in the day to help balance the books. For example, you may be aiming for 75 counts and usually eat:

Breakfast: 15/Snack: 5/Lunch: 20/Snack: 5/Dinner: 25/Treat: 5

If you go out for a 30 count dinner with a 10 count dessert and wine, then your day might be more like below, with 1 count (bonus) foods (like big salads and vegetable soups) helping you out on that day:

Breakfast: 10/Snack: 5/Lunch: 20/Dinner: 30/Treat: 10

You can see how the menu plans (right) increase or decrease the counts by simply changing the portion size or volume. Another way of increasing counts is to keep the portion size or volume the same and use an 'Add on' of, say, 5 counts. So if you are a 20 count breakfast person, you can choose a 15 count breakfast plan with, say, a small serve of cereal, and 'Add 5' toast and jam.

AS YOU GET STARTED, REMEMBER YOUR BODY STILL NEEDS ITS:

- ONE or more portions of lean meat, fish or other protein-rich food.
- TWO portions of fruit.
- THREE portions of low-fat dairy or other calcium-rich foods.
- FOUR-PLUS portions of cereals and starch foods, mostly wholegrain.
- FIVE or more portions of bonus vegetables, mostly low-starch ones.

As you learn this new way of living, remember that every day is a new day and it's important to keep focused on the solution rather than getting lost in the problem. Achieving a happy weight is about so much more than the food you eat—it's how, when and why you eat it. With all the new tools available to you and your own inherent wisdom, you are well on the road to success. Be kind to yourself. And good luck!

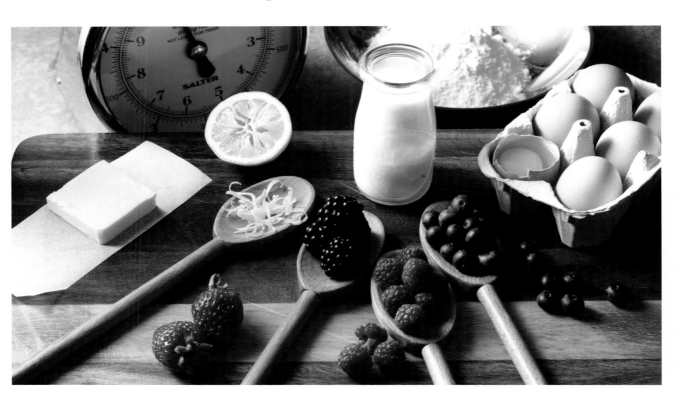

My mix-and-match menu plan

60 COUNT PLAN	75 COUNT PLAN	100 COUNT PLAN	110 COUNT PLAN

BREAKFAST

10 COUNT BREAKFAST	15 COUNT BREAKFAST	20 COUNT BREAKFAST	25 COUNT BREAKFAST
Cereal starter Choose: 1 cup (30g) wholegrain cereal OR ¼ cup (30g) muesli OR 2 breakfast biscuits OR 1 sachet instant oats *Serve with:* ½ cup low-fat (1.4%) milk 1 tsp sugar Black tea with dash of milk	*Cereal starter* Choose: 1½ cups (45g) wholegrain cereal OR ⅓ cup (45g) muesli OR 3 breakfast biscuits OR ⅓ cup dry rolled oats *Serve with:* ¾ cup low-fat milk 1 tsp sugar Black tea with dash of milk	*Cereal starter* Choose: 2 cups (60g) wholegrain cereal OR ½ cup (65g) muesli OR 4 breakfast biscuits OR ½ cup dry rolled oats *Serve with:* 1 cup low-fat milk 1 tsp sugar Black tea with dash of milk	*Cereal starter* *(Same as 100 count plan breakfast ➤)* Add on 5: 1 toast 1 scrape margarine Vegemite
Toast and coffee to go 1 thin slice grainy toast *Top with:* 1 scrape margarine and 1 tbsp fruit spread OR peanut butter OR cream cheese OR Vegemite PLUS 3* *Serve with:* NESCAFÉ Skim Cappuccino	*Toast and coffee to go* 1 thick slice grainy toast *Top with:* 2 scrapes margarine 1 tbsp fruit spread OR 1 scrape margarine and 1 tbsp peanut butter OR 1 scrape margarine and cream cheese *Serve with:* Small skinny Cappuccino	*Toast and coffee to go* 2 thick slices grainy toast *Top with:* 3 scrapes margarine and 2 tbsp Vegemite OR 2 tbsp fruit spread and 1 tbsp low-fat ricotta or cottage cheese *Serve with:* Small skinny cappuccino	*Toast and coffee to go* *(Same as 100 count plan breakfast ➤)* Add on 5: 1 cup (250ml) fruit juice
Fruit and yoghurt 1 fruit OR 1 cup homemade fruit salad *Serve with:* ½ tub (100g) low-fat yoghurt NESCAFÉ Skim Latte	*Fruit and yoghurt* 2 fruit OR 2 cups homemade fruit salad *Serve with:* ½ tub (100g) low-fat yoghurt Small skinny cappuccino	*Fruit and yoghurt* 2 fruit OR 2 cups homemade fruit salad *Serve with:* 1 tub (200g) low-fat sweetened yoghurt sprinkled with 1 tbsp dried fruit, seed or nut mix Black coffee	*Fruit and yoghurt* *(Same as 100 count plan breakfast ➤)* Add on 5: Dash of milk in coffee 1 small toasted waffle with 1 tsp topping
Time to cook 1 large (53g) egg poached, boiled or scrambled 1 thin slice toast with 1 scrape margarine *Serve with:* Tea with milk	*Time to cook* 1 large (53g) egg poached, boiled or scrambled 2 thin slices toast with 2 scrapes margarine *Serve with:* Tea with milk	*Time to cook* 2 medium (47g) eggs 2 thin slices toast with 2 scrapes margarine and 1 scrape marmalade *Serve with:* Tea with milk *PLUS 1 (e.g., teaspoon sugar)	*Time to cook* *(Same as 100 count plan breakfast ➤)* Add on 5: 1 cup orange and mango juice

*PLUS—When your counts fall short, you can pick something extra or save the counts for something like a piece of fruit or skinny cappuccino later in the day.

LUNCH

15 COUNT LUNCH	20 COUNT LUNCH	25 COUNT LUNCH	25 COUNT LUNCH
Cut and go sandwich 2 slices bread Spread 1 side (1 tsp margarine/1 tbsp hummus or mustard) 1 slice lean bone ham Salad leaves 1 fruit or small juice	*Cut and go sandwich* 2 slices bread Spread both sides (2 tsp margarine/2 tbsp hummus or mustard) 2 slices lean bone ham Salad leaves 1 fruit or small juice	*Cut and go sandwich* 1 long bread roll Spread both sides (2 tsp margarine) Dash mustard 2 slices lean bone ham Salad leaves 1 fruit or small juice	*Cut and go sandwich* 1 long bread roll Spread both sides (2 tsp margarine) Dash mustard 2 slices lean bone ham Salad leaves 1 fruit or small juice
Super salads 1 serve (40g) chicken/meat or small tin fish 1½ cups salad: grated carrot, lettuce, beans, baby tomato, etc. 1 slice light cheese 1 tbsp oil dressing 1 slice bread and margarine or 60g potato salad	*Super salads* 1 serve (40g) chicken/meat or small tin fish 1½ cups salad: grated carrot, lettuce, beans, baby tomato, etc. 1 slice light cheese 1 tbsp oil dressing 2 slices bread and margarine or 120g potato salad	*Super salads* 2 serves (80g) chicken/meat or medium tin fish 1½ cups salad: grated carrot, lettuce, beans, baby tomato, etc. 1 slice regular cheese 1 tbsp oil dressing 2 slices bread and margarine or 120g potato salad	*Super salads* 2 serves (80g) chicken/meat or medium tin fish 1½ cups salad: grated carrot, lettuce, beans, baby tomato, etc. 1 slice regular cheese 1 tbsp oil dressing 2 slices bread and margarine or 120g potato salad
Soup to sip Packet soup in a cup 1 small (30g) grain roll 1 scrape margarine 1 piece fruit Instant coffee with milk *PLUS 1	*Soup to sip* Packet soup in a cup 1 medium (65g) grain roll 2 scrapes margarine 1 piece fruit Instant coffee with milk	*Soup to sip* Packet soup in a cup 1 medium (65g) grain roll 2 scrapes margarine 1 piece fruit Instant coffee with milk *Add on 5:* 8 dried apple rings	*Soup to sip* Packet soup in a cup 1 medium (65g) grain roll 2 scrapes margarine 1 piece fruit Instant coffee with milk *Add on 5:* Handful of dried fruit
In the food hall or canteen 1 sushi roll or Salad sandwich with spread one side *Serve with:* Flavoured low fat milk (250ml/1 cup)	*In the food hall or canteen* 8 piece sushi tray or Pita wrap with ham, cheese and salad *Serve with:* Water or diet soda	*In the food hall or canteen* 2 sushi rolls or Noodle box (small) with chicken and vegetables *Serve with:* Flavoured milk (300ml)	*In the food hall or canteen* 2 sushi rolls or Noodle box (small) with chicken and vegetables *Serve with:* Flavoured milk (300ml)
SNACKS 10 COUNTS	SNACKS 10 COUNTS	SNACKS 15 COUNTS	SNACKS 15 COUNTS
Choose: 1 or 2 snacks from the table on page 220 to equal 10 counts during the day	Choose: 1 or 2 snacks from the table on page 220 to equal 10 counts during the day	Choose: 1, 2 or 3 snacks from the table on page 220 to equal 15 counts during the day	Choose: 1, 2 or 3 snacks from the table on page 220 to equal 15 counts during the day

DINNER

20 COUNT DINNER	25 COUNT DINNER	30 COUNT DINNER	35 COUNT DINNER
Meat and 3 veg Small serve meat (100g) ½ plate bonus veggies 2 medium potatoes OR 1 cup cooked pasta or rice	*Meat and 3 veg* Small serve meat (100g) ½ plate bonus veggies 2 medium potatoes OR 1 cup cooked pasta or rice *Add 5:* 2 scoops of no-added-sugar ice cream	*Meat and 3 veg* Small serve meat (100g) ½ plate bonus veggies 2 medium potatoes OR 1 cup cooked pasta or rice *Add 10:* 2 scoops of low-fat ice cream ½ cup fruit, canned or stewed, no added sugar	*Meat and 3 veg* Medium serve meat (150g) ½ plate bonus veggies 2 medium potatoes OR 1 cup cooked pasta or rice *Add 10:* 2 scoops low-fat ice cream ½ cup fruit, canned or stewed, no added sugar
One-dish dinner 1 small serve mince or chopped meat (85g raw weight) Add: tomato pasta sauce and chopped vegetables (see easy bolognaise, page 121) *Serve with:* ½ cup spaghetti or noodles	*One-dish dinner* 1 small serve mince or chopped meat (85g raw weight) Add: tomato pasta sauce and chopped vegetables (see easy bolognaise, page 121) *Serve with:* 1 cup spaghetti or noodles *Plus:* Fresh platter of fruit slices equal to 1 fresh fruit	*One-dish dinner* 1 medium serve mince or chopped meat (125g raw weight) Add: tomato pasta sauce and chopped vegetables (see easy bolognaise, page 121) *Serve with:* 1 cup spaghetti or noodles *Plus:* Fresh platter of fruit slices equal to 2 fresh fruit	*One-dish dinner* 1 medium serve mince or chopped meat (125g raw weight) Add: tomato pasta sauce and chopped vegetables (see easy bolognaise, page 121) *Serve with:* 1½ cups spaghetti or noodles *Plus:* Fresh platter of fruit slices equal to 2 fresh fruit
Curry and salad 1 serve beef curry with rice (see recipe, page 100) Chopped tomato with mint	*Curry and salad* 1 serve beef curry with rice (see recipe, page 100) Chopped tomato with mint *Add 5:* ⅓ cup cucumber raita 1 tbsp mango chutney	*Curry and salad* 1 serve beef curry with rice (see recipe, page 100) Chopped tomato with mint *Add 10:* ⅓ cup cucumber raita 1 tbsp mango chutney 2 large pappadums	*Curry and salad* 1⅓ serve beef curry with rice (see recipe, page 100, and divide by 5 instead of 6) Chopped tomato with mint *Add 10:* ⅓ cup cucumber raita 1 tbsp mango chutney 2 large pappadums
Takeaway option Takeaway Chinese beef combination noodles (1 cup)	*Takeaway option* Takeaway Chinese beef combination noodles (1 cup) *Add 5:* 1 bowl of lychees	*Takeaway option* Takeaway Chinese beef combination noodles (1 cup) *Add 10:* 1 bowl of lychees 2 scoops non-fat gelato	*Takeaway option* Takeaway Chinese beef combination noodles (1 cup) *Add 15:* 1 bowl of lychees 2 scoops non-fat gelato 1 glass wine (150ml)
Stir fry Seafood and basil stir fry (see recipe on page 138) ½ cup boiled rice	*Stir fry* Seafood and basil stir fry (see recipe on page 138) 1 cup boiled rice	*Stir fry* Seafood and basil stir fry (see recipe on page 138) 1 cup boiled rice *Add 5:* 1 tub (125g) low-fat Frûche fromage frais	*Stir fry* Seafood and basil stir fry (see recipe on page 138) 1 cup boiled rice *Add 10:* 2 scoops regular ice cream

MY MIX-AND-MATCH MENU PLAN

TREATS 5 COUNTS	TREATS 5 COUNTS	TREATS 10 COUNTS	TREATS 10 COUNTS
Choose a small 5 count treat from the table below per day if you like to, or add another snack instead	Choose a small 5 count treat from the table below per day if you like to, or add another snack instead	Choose up to 10 counts of treats from the table below per day, or include another snack instead	Choose up to 10 counts of treats from the table below per day, or include another snack instead

SNACKS, TREATS AND DRINKS

SNACKS AND DRINKS
0–4 COUNTS

0 count:
Water
Diet soft drink
Vegetable sticks

1 count:
Black coffee or tea with
  dash of milk

2 counts:
Vegetable sticks with salsa
  or low-fat hummus
Punnet of strawberries
100g diet yoghurt
Sachet NESCAFÉ Skim Latte
  or Cappuccino

3 counts:
1 small fruit
Bunch of 20 grapes
½ cup canned fruit, no
  added sugar
4 small pieces dried fruit
2 cups popcorn

4 counts:
1 average piece fruit,
200ml fruit juice,
200g diet yoghurt,
100g low-fat fruit yoghurt
Skinny cappuccino/latte
  (regular size)
BILLABONG ice cream

SNACKS AND DRINKS
5-10 COUNTS

5 counts:
1 slice reduced-fat cheese
  with 2 Cruskit crackers
1 toast with margarine
  and Vegemite
Handful of nuts
  (e.g., 15 almonds)
COUNTRY CUP soup

6 counts:
Muesli bar, wholegrain
Fruit bread or crumpet
  with margarine
½ avocado, medium
Box of sultanas

7 counts:
1 glass MILO with skim milk
Scone with margarine
Cappuccino, full cream
  (250ml)

9 counts:
Packet nuts (30g)
Large fruit juice (400ml)
200g reduced fat fruit
  yoghurt

10 counts:
Fruit smoothie

11 counts:
Iced coffee/chocolate
Large caramel chai latte
  (300–400ml)

SMALL TREATS
2-9 COUNTS

2 counts:
1 lemonade ICY POLE
1 fruit slice biscuit
1 stick liquorice
1 piece chocolate (9g)

3 counts:
1 fruit pillow biscuit
1 scoop PETERS light and
  creamy ice cream

4 counts:
1 shortbread biscuit
1 small muffin (30g)
1 tbsp double cream
1 SKINNY COW ice cream

5 counts:
1 chocolate biscuit
1 party pie
1 Dixie Cup ice cream
2 snakes
6 marshmallows
12 LIFE SAVERS
12 jelly beans

6 counts:
1 chips, multipack
1 slice (40g) sponge
  swiss roll

7 counts:
1 small cupcake, iced
1 soft-serve ice cream
1 row plain chocolate

8 counts:
1 CHOC WEDGE ice cream

9 counts:
1 scoop premium ice cream

TREATS AND DESSERTS
FOR SPECIAL OCCASIONS
10+ COUNTS

10 counts:
1 slice banana bread or cake
1 piece baklava

11 counts:
1 chocolate brownie
1 DRUMSTICK ice cream

12 counts:
1 finger bun
1 plain cinnamon doughnut
50g bag potato chips

13 counts:
1 slice pavlova and cream
1 medium piece vanilla slice

14 counts:
1 small cup hot chips
1 chocolate HEAVEN ice
  cream

15 counts:
1 slice chocolate bavarian

DRINK COUNTS
Soda/mineral water = 0
1 nip spirits = 3
1 small glass (120ml) dry
  white wine = 4
1 nip spirits with mixer
  (e.g., rum and coke) = 6
1 light beer (375ml) = 5
Coke/lemonade (375ml) = 7
1 full-strength beer
  (375ml) = 7

How we counted the counts

It's good to remember:
1 count = approximately
87 kilojoules, or about
20 calories.

If you study the food packs over the breakfast table, you may have already worked out how the counts have been calculated. The %DI on the front of the majority of food products is a simple calculation made using a product's energy (kilojoule or calorie) level per serve. Essentially, one count equals approximately 87 kilojoules, or about 20 calories.

In the ready-reckoner that follows, we calculated the average counts for a wide range of popular foods. To put this ready-reckoner together we trekked through supermarkets recording counts off the front of packs, we checked and cross-referenced common databases, and when there were similar foods we calculated an average. We rounded the counts up or down and haven't included half-counts, and we encourage you to do the same—be careful tracking your counts but don't get too anxious about the minute detail. Remember, kilojoules and calories in food can vary in their composition in nature, and can also differ in how our individual bodies utilise them. This makes kilojoules a very inexact science to begin with. An estimation is all that is required to make counting work well and to bring the awareness and insight you need to manage your weight better by making more informed choices.

So be curious but not fanatical about the counts. Search out lighter options or change the serving size to lower the total counts you eat. The difference in 1 count will have little impact, but 10 or 20 will! When buying your favourite foods, check the labels to see if different manufacturers or formulation modifications have changed the counts quoted here. If you're an adventurous eater and the %DI is not recorded on the pack or in our ready-reckoner, call the company's consumer services line. Most companies have a toll-free number and employ helpful staff to provide you with additional information. After all, how can they expect you to use their product if they don't provide you with all the details you need to use it easily?

Alternatively, if you find you only have the kilojoule level declared on the pack or you wish to make a recipe that has the kilojoules or calories per serve but no count tally, it's easy for you to work out your own counts—just grab a pad and pen (or calculator) and start adding. An example below is a small box of sultanas which says it has 418kJ per pack

Sultana box: 418kJ per pack

Calculator method:
418kJ ÷ 87kJ
= 4.8 (round up to)
≈ 5 counts

Mental arithmetic method:
1. 418kJ ÷ 4
≈ 100 Calories

2. 100 Calories ÷ 20 Calories
≈ 5 counts

NOTE: To convert kilojoules to counts divide by 87 (87 kJ=1 count)

NOTE 1. To convert kilojoules easily to Calories divide by 4 (1 Calorie=4.2kJ)
NOTE 2. To convert Calories easily to counts divide by 20 (20.8 Calories = 1 count)

KEY: ÷ means divide and ≈ means approximately

Ready-reckoner

Bakery

This section includes all bakery-type products, such as biscuits (sweet and savoury), crispbread, crackers, bread, rolls and buns, crumpets, muffins, pancakes, cakes, desserts, pies and pastries. We have also included some baking and pastry ingredients.

BISCUITS, CRISPBREAD AND CRACKERS, SAVOURY

Biscuit, flavoured shapes, 10 biscuits (20g)	5
Biscuit, mini wholegrain, 17 biscuits (20g)	4
Corn cake, 1 cake (6g)	1
Crispbread, rye, 2 pieces (20g)	3
Crispbread, wholemeal wheat flour, 2 pieces (12g)	2
Crispbread, with seeds, 2 pieces (20g)	4
Lavosh, unflavoured, 2 biscuits (14g)	3
Melba toast, 2 biscuits (1g)	1
Pastry twist, cheese flavoured, 3 biscuits (27g)	6
Rice cake, 1 thin cake (6g)	1
Rice cake, 1 thick cake (10g)	2
Rice crackers, wholegrain, 3 crackers (5g)	1
Watercracker style, 5 crackers (15g)	3

BISCUITS, SWEET

Anzac biscuit, 1 biscuit (16g)	4
Biscotti with roasted almonds, 1 biscuit (10g)	2
Biscuit with chocolate chip or chocolate coating, 1 biscuit (20g)	5
Biscuit with dried fruit and nut, 1 large biscuit (33g)	8
Biscuit with dried fruit, 1 biscuit (10g)	2
Biscuit with icing, 1 biscuit (10g)	2
Biscuit with mint filling and chocolate coating, 1 biscuit (15g)	4
Chocolate biscuit (similar to Tim Tam), 1 biscuit (19g)	5
Fortune cookie, 1 cookie (8g)	2
Ginger flavoured, 1 biscuit (13g)	3
Jam, marshmallow or cream filling, 1 biscuit (20g)	4
Macaroon, 1 biscuit (20g)	5
Oatmeal or wheatmeal, 1 biscuit (8g)	2
Plain or flavoured, digestive-style, 1 biscuit (8g)	2
Rice cake, carob coated, 1 biscuit (25g)	4
Shortbread, 1 biscuit (17g)	4
Sponge finger style, 1 biscuit (12g)	2
Wafer biscuit with filling, 1 biscuit (6g)	1

BREAD ROLLS AND BUNS

Bagel, large (85g)	12
Bagel, medium (55g)	7
Bagel, small (30g)	4
Bread roll, mixed grain, large (83g)	9
Bread roll, white, hamburger style (74g)	9
Bread roll, white, hot dog style (62g)	8
Bread roll, white, jumbo size (82g)	10
Bread roll, white, large (45g)	5
Bread roll, white, small (30g)	3
Bread roll, wholegrain, large (100g)	11
Bread roll, wholegrain, medium (65g)	7
Bread roll, wholegrain, small (30g)	4
Bread roll, long, wholegrain, small (90g)	10
Bread roll, long, wholegrain, large (170g)	19

BREAD, SLICED

Bakery bread, white, 1 thin slice (30g)	4
Gluten-free bread, mixed grain or white, 1 slice (26g)	3
Grain bread with barley, 1 heavy slice (49g)	6
Homemade bread from bread mix, 1 slice (48g)	6
Mixed grain or multigrain bread, 1 thick slice (45g)	5
Mixed grain or multigrain bread, 1 thin slice (30g)	3
Mixed grain bread, 1 double-thick slice (70g)	8
Rye bread, dark, 1 slice (41g)	4
Rye bread, light, 1 slice (43g)	5
Sourdough bread, 1 slice (40g)	5
Soy linseed bread, 1 thick slice (40g)	5
White bread, 1 thin slice (30g)	4
Wholemeal bread with grain and/or seeds, 1 thick slice (45g)	5
Wholemeal bread with grain and/or seeds, 1 thin slice (34g)	4

Wholemeal bread with seeds and oats, 1 thin slice (34g)	4
Wholemeal bread, 1 double-thick slice (70g)	8
Wholemeal bread, 1 thin slice (27g)	3
Wholemeal bread, 1 toasting slice (40g)	4

SPECIALTY BREADS

Bruschetta/ciabatta Italian-style bread, 1 medium slice (27g)	3
Chapatti, no added fat, 1 chapatti (35g)	3
Damper, 1 wedge (60g)	7
Focaccia, plain, small piece (50g)	7
Foccacia, plain, large piece (¼ of the bread) (88g)	10
French stick (baguette), 1.5cm slice (12g)	2
Garlic bread, 1 slice with butter (23g)	4
Herb bread with butter, 1 big slice (45g)	7
Lebanese bread, white, 1 whole (84g)	12
Lebanese bread, wholemeal, 1 whole (100g)	15
Naan bread, 1 whole (130g)	18
Naan bread, ½ slice (65g)	9
Pagnotta, Italian-style bread, small slice (19g)	2
Pita pocket bread, small (28g)	4
Pita pocket bread, large (60g)	8
Pizza base, ¼ pizza base (42g)	6
Pappadams, microwaved, 2 small (8g)	1
Pappadams, microwaved, 2 large (19g)	2
Pumpernickel, 1 slice (5g)	5
Taco shell, from cornflour, plain, 1 shell (13g)	3
Tortilla, burrito, 1 burrito (40g)	7
Tortilla, plain, 1 small tortilla (25g)	4
Tortilla, plain, 1 large tortilla (50g)	8
Turkish pide bread, ¼ large roll (100g)	11
Wrap, gluten free, 1 wrap (42g)	7
Wrap, light, 1 wrap (25g)	3
Wrap, wholemeal, large (57g)	10
Wrap, wholemeal, small (40g)	7

CRUMPETS, FRUIT BREADS, MUFFINS AND PANCAKES

Croissant, cheese and ham filled, 1 croissant (90g)	14
Croissant, plain, fresh, 1 croissant (67g)	12
Croissant, 1 frozen (50g)	9
Croissant, 1 large (75g)	13
Crumpet, white, 1 round crumpet (50g)	4
Crumpet, wholemeal, 1 round crumpet (50g)	4
Fruit loaf, 1 thin slice (33g)	4
Fruit loaf, dense, 1 slice (45g)	6
Hot cross bun, 1 bun (75g)	11
Muffin, English, spicy fruit, 1 muffin (67g)	8
Muffin, English, white, wholemeal or multigrain, 1 muffin (67g)	8
Muffin, English with cheese and egg, fast-food style, 1 muffin (100g)	13
Muffin, English with cheese, egg and bacon, fast-food style, 1 muffin (132g)	17
Muffin, average, 1 large (100g)	17
Muffin, average, 1 medium (60g)	10
Muffin, average, 1 small (30g)	5
Pancake, large, 12cm (83g)	11
Pancake, medium, 10cm (40g)	5
Pancake, small, 8cm (25g)	3
Pancake, bought, 1 large (60g)	7
Pikelet, 1 homemade (20g)	2
Pikelet, 1 bought (25g)	3
Raisin bread, 1 slice (30g)	4
Scone, plain, 1 scone (40g)	5
Scone, white, with cheese, 1 scone (85g)	13
Scone with jam and cream, fast-food style, 1 scone (85g)	23
Waffle, 1 plain large (75g)	12

CAKES AND DESSERTS

Baklava, 1 piece (50g)	10
Banana bread, 1 slice (60g)	9
Bun finger with icing, 1 bun (85g)	12
Cake, apple, un-iced, 1 slice (88g)	14
Cake, banana, 1 slice (60g)	10
Cake, black forest, layered, cream filled, 1 slice (88g)	15
Cake, carrot, iced, 1 slice (88g)	16
Cake, cheesecake, biscuit base, cream cheese topping, 1 slice (140g)	23
Cake, chocolate mud, iced, 1 slice (100g)	21
Cake, cupcake, iced, small (40g)	7
Cake, fruit, light style, un-iced, 1 slice (88g)	15
Cake, plain or butter cake, un-iced, 1 slice (88g)	15
Cake, sponge Swiss roll, 1 slice (40g)	6
Cake, sponge, plain, unfilled, un-iced, 1 slice (88g)	13

Chocolate bavarian, 1 slice (93g)	15
Chocolate brownie, 1 slice (56g)	11
Chocolate éclair, 1 large (120g)	23
Crumble, apple, berry or rhubarb, 1 serve (191g)	15
Custard tart, 1 tart (140g)	17
Custard, low fat, ½ cup (100)	5
Custard, rice, 1 tub (150g)	8
Custard, traditional, ½ cup (100g)	6
Doughnut, custard filled, 1 doughnut (112g)	16
Doughnut, dusted with cinnamon and sugar, 1 doughnut (70g)	12
Doughnut, jam filled, sugar coated, 1 doughnut (86g)	15
Friand, 1 friand (60g)	8
Gingerbread, iced, 1 biscuit (36g)	6
Jam rolette, 1 piece (28g)	4
Jelly, ½ cup (120g)	4
Lamington, 1 medium (80g)	12
Meringue, 3 small kisses (5g)	1
Mousse, Bavarian cream, 1 serve (108g)	18
Mousse, chocolate mud, 1 cup (180g)	17
Pavlova with fruit and cream, 1 slice (120g)	13
Pie, apple, 1 small pie (150g)	17
Pie, lemon meringue, 1 slice (113g)	15
Pie, pecan, 1 slice (113g)	22
Pudding, bread and butter, baked, 1 serve (90g)	7
Pudding, rice, 1 cup (238g)	17
Pudding, self-saucing, chocolate flavour, prepared from dry mix, 1 serve (90g)	9
Pudding, sticky date, 1 serve (100g)	18
Rum ball truffle, 1 rum ball (9g)	2
Scroll, apple and custard, 1 scroll (145g)	23
Slice, caramel, 1 slice (80g)	19
Slice, dried fruit filling, iced, 1 large slice (219g)	31
Slice, jelly, 1 serve (90g)	13
Slice, marshmallow, 1 serve (46g)	10
Slice, muesli, wholemeal with chocolate chips, 1 bar (120g)	25
Slice, rice bubble, 1 serve (56g)	11
Slice, vanilla custard filling, iced, 1 slice (173g)	17
Slice, vanilla, 1 medium (130g)	13
Soufflé, berry, 1 serve (150g),	18

PIES AND PASTRIES

Curry puff, beef, deep-fried in oil, 1 puff (50g)	6
Meat pie, 1 single (175g)	22
Meat pie, party size (mini), 1 pie (38g)	5
Pastry, meat and nut filling (lady fingers), Lebanese style, 1 piece (42g)	6
Pastry, spinach filling, Lebanese style, 1 piece (42g)	6
Pasty, vegetable and meat, ready to eat, 1 pasty (188g)	23
Pie, meat, individual size, ready to eat, 1 pie (174g)	20
Pie, vegetable, 1 pie (390g)	36
Quiche, homemade, 1 slice (150g)	19
Quiche, small (115g)	14
Sausage roll, 1 large (130g)	18
Sausage roll, 1 party size (mini) (35g)	6
Spring roll, 1 spring roll (170g)	19
vol-au-vents, unfilled, 1 small case (5g)	1
vol-au-vents, unfilled, 1 large case (13g)	3

BAKING AND PASTRY INGREDIENTS

Breadcrumbs, ¼ cup (30g)	4
Cocoa powder, 1 tbsp (7g)	1
Cornflour, 1 cup (135g)	23
Croutons, ¼ cup (10g)	2
Flour, gluten free, self-raising, 1 cup (140g)	24
Flour, rice, 1 cup (165g)	26
Flour, rye, wholemeal, 1 cup (110g)	15
Flour, soy, low fat, 1 cup (140g)	24
Flour, wheat, white, plain or self-raising, 1 cup (140g)	24
Flour, wheat, wholemeal, plain or self-raising, 1 cup (140g)	22
Icing (without the cake), 1 tbsp (20g)	5
Pastry, choux, baked, unfilled, 1 profiterole case (8g)	1
Quinoa, wholegrain or flour, 1 cup (180g)	31
Sugar, caster, 4 tsp (16g)	3
Sugar, white, 1 tsp (4g)	1

Breakfast cereals

This section includes a range of breakfast cereals found on most supermarket shelves.

Cereal bites (UNCLE TOBYS Fruit Bites), 1 cup (35g)	6
CHEERIOS, 1 cup (30g)	5
Corn Flakes, 1 cup (30g)	5
UNCLE TOBYS PLUS FIBRE LIFT cereal, small bag (35g)	6
Mixed cereal (oat, corn, rice, barley), extruded, 1 cup (40g)	7
Muesli, toasted, ⅓ cup (45g)	9
Muesli, untoasted or natural style, ⅓ cup (45g)	8
Oat flake breakfast biscuit, 1 biscuit (21g)	4
Oat bran, unprocessed, 1 tbsp (11g)	2
Oats, flavoured, sachet (30g)	6
Oats, traditional, ¼ cup	5
Porridge, rolled oats prepared with full-fat milk, 1 cup (260g)	14
Porridge, rolled oats prepared with reduced-fat milk, 1 cup (260g)	11
Porridge, rolled oats prepared with skim milk, 1 cup (260g)	10
Porridge, rolled oats, prepared with water, 1 cup (260g)	7
Puffed whole wheat, 1 cup (30g)	5
Puffed corn, 1 cup (30g)	5
Puffed or popped rice, 1 cup (30g)	6
Rice porridge (congee), cooked, 1 cup (242g)	4
WEETIES, 1 cup (30g)	5
Wheat, extruded, chocolate coated, 1 cup (40g)	8
Wheat bran, unprocessed, ½ cup (31g)	3
Wheat bran, processed straws, ¾ cup (45g)	7
Wheat bran flakes, sweetened, 1 cup (40g)	6
Wheat flake breakfast biscuit, 1 biscuit (15g)	3
Wheat flakes with fruit pieces, ¾ cup (45g)	8
Wheat germ, ½ tbsp (5g)	1

Canned meals

This section includes several varieties of tinned baked beans and spaghetti.

Baked beans, canned, 1 small can (130g)	5
Baked beans in tomato sauce, ½ cup (150g)	6
Baked beans in ham sauce, ½ cup (150g)	8
Spaghetti in cheese and tomato sauce, canned (large 440g can)	16
Spaghetti in cheese and tomato sauce, canned (medium 225g can)	8
Spaghetti in cheese and tomato sauce, canned (small 130g can)	5
Spaghetti in meat sauce, canned (large 420g can)	15
Spaghetti in meat sauce, canned (small 140g can)	5
Spaghetti in tomato sauce, canned (large 420g can)	12
Spaghetti in tomato sauce, canned (medium 220g can)	6
Spaghetti in tomato sauce, canned (small 120g can)	4
Steak and onions, canned (large 425g)	15

Condiments

This section includes products such as dips, dressings, gravies, sauces and spreads.

Beetroot dip, 2 tbsp (40g)	2
Cream cheese-based dip, flavoured (e.g., French onion), 1 tbsp (20g)	2
Hummus, regular, 1 tbsp (20g)	2
Hummus, chunky style (with nuts), 1 tbsp (20g)	4
French onion dip, 1 tbsp (20g)	2
Sour cream-based dip, light, 1 tbsp (20g)	2
Tahini, 1 tbsp (25g)	8
Tzatziki, 2 tbsp (40g)	2

Dressing, avocado, 1 tbsp (20g)	2
Dressing, Caesar, 1 tbsp (20g)	5
Dressing, coleslaw, regular, 1 tbsp (20g)	4
Dressing, fat free, 2 tsp (10ml)	0
Dressing, French, regular, 1 tbsp (20g)	3
Dressing, honey mustard, 1 tbsp (20g)	2

Dressing, Italian, regular, 1 tbsp (20g)	3
Dressing, salad, oil and vinegar, homemade, 1 tbsp (20g)	4
Dressing, thousand island, regular, 1 tbsp (20g)	4
Vinaigrette, 1 tbsp (20g)	3

GRAVIES

Gravy, homemade, 3 tbsp (60ml)	3
Gravy, prepared from dry mix, 3 tbsp (60ml)	1

OTHER

Grainy mustard, 1 tsp (5g)	0
Horseradish cream, 2 tsp (10g)	1
Light (97% fat-free) mayonnaise, 1 tbsp (30g)	1
Mayonnaise, full fat, 2 tsp (10g)	4
Mayonnaise, full fat, 1 tbsp (20g)	7
Pickle, BRANSTON, 1 serve (20g)	1
Pickles, mustard, sweet, 1 tbsp (22g)	2
Relish, corn, 1 tbsp (19g)	2

SAUCES

Barbecue sauce, 1 tbsp (20g)	2
Béarnaise sauce, 1 tbsp (20g)	2
Black bean sauce, Asian style, 1 tbsp (20g)	1
Butter chicken sauce, Indian style, packet mix, 1 packet (35g)	2
Cheese sauce, 1 tbsp (25g)	2
Chilli sauce, Asian style, 1 tbsp (20g)	2
Chutney, 1 tbsp (25g)	2
Cranberry jelly, 1 tbsp (20g)	2
Cranberry sauce, 1 tbsp (20g)	2
Curry sauce, 1 tbsp (20g)	1
Fish sauce, 1 tbsp (20g)	0
Hollandaise sauce, 1 tbsp (20g)	5
Mint jelly, 1 tbsp (20g)	3
Mint sauce, 1 tbsp (18g)	1
Mushroom sauce, 1 cup (250g)	3
Oyster sauce, 1 tbsp (20g)	1
Pasta sauce, cream based, ½ cup (125g)	6
Pepper sauce with gravy, 1 cup (250g)	3
Pesto, 1 tbsp (20g)	2
Plum sauce, Asian style, 1 tbsp (20g)	2
Rogan josh sauce, 1 tbsp (20g)	1
Satay peanut sauce, 1 tbsp (20g)	2
Soy sauce, 1 tbsp (21g)	0

Sweet and sour sauce, ¼ cup (70g)	6
Taramasalata, 2 tbsp (40g)	5
Tartar sauce, 1 tbsp (20g)	2
Tomato salsa, fresh, 2 tbsp (50g)	0
Tomato salsa, bought, 4 tbsp (100g)	2
Tomato sauce, 1 tbsp (20g)	1
Worcestershire sauce, 1 tbsp (24g)	1

SPREADS

Anchovy spread, ½ small jar (25g)	2
Cheese spread, 1 tbsp (21g)	3
Chocolate/nut spread, 1 tbsp (20g)	5
Honey, 1 tsp (6g)	1
Hummus, *see* Condiments	
Jam or marmalade, 2 tsp (15g)	2
Olive tapenade, 1 tbsp (20g)	4
Peanut butter, smooth or crunchy, 1 tbsp (20g)	6
Peanut butter, light, 1 tbsp (20g)	5
Yeast-extract spread, 1 tsp (6g)	1

Confectionery

This section includes both chocolate and sugar confectionery.

CHOCOLATE

Bar, average fun-sized chocolate bar, filled, 1 bar (13g)	3
Bar, caramel centre, milk chocolate, 1 bar (47g)	10
Bar, carob, 1 row (19g)	5
Bar, cherry and coconut centre, dark chocolate, 1 bar (55g)	11
Bar, chocolate and cookie pieces, white chocolate, 1 bar (55g)	13
Bar, chocolate and peppermint crisps, milk chocolate, 1 bar (35g)	9
Bar, chocolate and rice crisps, milk chocolate, 1 bar (55g)	13
Bar, chocolate and whipped nougat centre, milk chocolate, 1 bar (25g)	5
Bar, chocolate (similar to AERO), 1 bar (20g)	5
Bar, coconut cream centre, milk chocolate, 1 bar (19g)	4
Bar, fudge centre, milk chocolate, 1 bar (47g)	10
Bar, honeycomb centre, chocolate, 1 bar (50g)	11
Bar, milk chocolate with nougat and almond pieces, 1 bar (47g)	12

Bar, nougat and caramel centre, milk chocolate, 1 bar (47g)	9
Bar, nougat, caramel and peanut centre, milk chocolate, 1 bar (60g)	12
Bar, nougat, milk chocolate, 1 bar (47g)	9
Bar, peanuts, wafer, caramel and rice crisps, milk chocolate, 1 bar (50g)	12
Bar, rice cereal and peanut, chocolate, 1 bar (35g)	8
Bar, wafer and caramel layers, milk chocolate, 1 bar (30g)	7
Bar, wafer and chocolate cream centre or caramel, milk chocolate, 1 bar (40g)	10
Bar, wafer and fudge centre, milk chocolate, 1 bar (47g)	11
Bar, wafer, caramel and peanut, chocolate, Snickers or Picnic style, 1 bar (50g)	12
Bar, wafer or biscuit and chocolate cream centre, milk chocolate, 1 bar (30g)	7
Chocolate or chocolate bar, filled, 1 piece (6.6g)	1
Chocolate, coated bar style, 1 bar (47g)	10
Chocolate, dark, 2 squares (22.5g)	6
Chocolate, dark with roasted almonds, 2 squares (22.5g)	6
Dried fruit and nut mix, milk chocolate or yoghurt coated, 10 pieces (10g)	2
Dried fruit, nut and chocolate mix, 10 pieces (10g)	2
Macadamia, milk chocolate coated, 10 pieces (29g)	9
Peanut, milk chocolate coated, 10 pieces (12g)	3
Rum balls, chocolate flavour, 1 serve (16g)	3
Truffle, chocolate with coconut, 1 piece (13g)	3

SUGAR SWEETS

Caramels, soft and hard varieties, 1 piece	1
Fudge, 1 piece (20g)	4
Ginger, crystallised, sweetened and preserved, 1 piece (5g)	1
Halvah, plain, 5 x 1cm cubes (6g)	1
Honeycomb, plain, 1 piece (18g)	3
Liquorice allsorts, 1 piece (7g)	1
Liquorice, large twists, 3 sticks (60g)	10
Liquorice, plain, 1 piece (13g)	2
Marshmallow, chocolate and coconut-coated (snowball), 1 snowball (26g)	5
Marshmallow, plain or flavoured, 5 pieces (30g)	5
Marzipan, almond paste, ¼ cup (60g)	12
Nougat, honey and almond, 1 bar (40g)	6
Sherbet, 1 packet (14g)	2
Sugar sweets, all types, chocolate-coated, 10 pieces (30g)	6
Sugar sweets, boiled, 1 piece (5g)	1
Sugar sweets, jelly varieties, 1 piece (6g)	1
Sugar sweets, mint flavoured, hard and chewy, 5 pieces (20g)	4
Sugar sweets, yoghurt-coated apricot, 1 piece (18g)	3
Turkish delight, 1 piece (18g)	3

Dairy and alternatives

This section includes cheeses, milks and eggs, as well as some of their dairy alternatives.

CHEESE

Blue vein, 1 wedge (22g)	4
Camembert or brie, 1 small wedge (30g)	4
Cheddar, extra light (50%), 1 slice (21g)	3
Cheddar, light, grated, cup (40g)	6
Cheddar, reduced fat (~25%), 1 slice (21g)	3
Cheddar, regular, 1 slice (21g)	4
Cheese spread, 1 tbsp (21g)	3
Cheese stick/wedge, 1 piece (20g)	3
Colby style, 1 slice (27g)	5
Cottage cheese, creamed, unflavoured, 1 cup (230g)	13
Cottage cheese, reduced fat, 1 tbsp (20g)	1
Cream cheese, 1 tbsp (20g)	3
Cream cheese, extra light, 1 tbsp (20g)	1
Cream cheese, light (~15% fat), 1 tbsp (20g)	2
Cream cheese, reduced fat (~25% fat), 1 tbsp (20g)	3
Edam, 1 slice (27g)	5
Feta, 4 cubes (60g)	8
Feta, reduced fat, 4 cubes (60g)	7
Fromage frais/Frûche, low fat, 1 tub (125g)	5
Goat cheese, 1 slice (27g)	3
Gouda, 1 slice (27g)	5
Haloumi, 1 slice (27g)	3
Havarti style, 1 slice (27g)	5
Mozzarella, 1 cup (119g)	18
Parmesan, 4 tbsp (30g)	6

Ricotta cheese, reduced fat (5%), 1 tbsp (30g)	1
Ricotta cheese, regular (10% fat), ½ cup (140g)	9
Soy cheese, ½ cup (82g)	14
Swiss cheese, 1 slice (27g)	5
MILK (1 cup = 250ml)	
Buttermilk, cultured, 2% fat, 1 cup	7
Cream *see* Eggs, fats, oils and cream	
Custard *see* Cakes and desserts	
Drink, probiotic, contains milk solids and sugar, 1 bottle (65g)	2
Drink, probiotic, contains milk solids and sugar, reduced sugar, 1 bottle (65g)	1
Flavoured milk *see* Drinks	
Milk, evaporated, regular, 1 cup	18
Milk, evaporated, skim (<0.5% fat), 1 cup	10
Milk, extra creamy (>4% fat), 1 cup	9
Milk, full cream (3.6%), 1 cup	8
Milk, goat, 1 cup	6
Milk, low fat (1.4%), 1 cup	6
Milk, oat, 1 cup	3
Milk, powder, goat, 1 tbsp (8.4g)	2
Milk, powder, regular, 1 tbsp (8.4g)	2
Milk, powder, skim, 1 tbsp (8g)	1
Milk, powder, whey, 1 cup (153g)	26
Milk, reduced fat (2%), 1 cup	7
Milk, rice, 1 cup	6
Milk, sheep, 1 cup	13
Milk, skim (0.1%), 1 cup	5
Milk, soy, fat free, 1 cup	4
Milk, soy, reduced fat, 1 cup	5
Milk, soy, regular, flavoured or plain, 1 cup	8
Milk, sweetened, condensed, regular, 1 cup	50
Milk, sweetened, condensed, skim (~0.2% fat), 1 cup	43

YOGHURT

Soy yoghurt, regular fat (~3%), 1 tub (208g)	9
Yoghurt, diet, 1 tub (200g)	4
Yoghurt, frozen, low fat, 1 scoop (50g)	4
Yoghurt, full cream, 1 tub (200g)	10
Yoghurt, Greek style, plain, 1 tub (208g)	14
Yoghurt, low fat (<0.5%), added sugar, 1 tub (200g)	8
Yoghurt, natural, reduced fat (~2%), 1 tub (200g)	9
Yoghurt, fruit, reduced fat, 1 tub (200g)	10

Drinks

This section includes all type of drinks, including alcohol, flavoured milk, coffee, tea, juice, cordial, waters, smoothies, soft drinks, and energy, sports and breakfast drinks.

ALCOHOL

Beer, full strength (4.9% alc.), 1 can (375ml)	7
Beer, original pale ale (4.5% alc.), 1 can (375ml)	6
Beer, premium (5% alc.), 1 can (375ml)	7
Beer, premium lager, low carb (4.6% alc.), 1 bottle (355ml)	5
Beer, premium light (2.6–2.9% alc.), 1 can (375ml)	5
Cider, original (5% alc), 1 bottle (355ml)	9
Cocktails, cosmopolitan, 1 cocktail, 250ml	7
Cocktails, mojito, 1 cocktail, 250ml	7
Cocktails, margarita, 1 cocktail, 250ml	5
Cocktails, pina colada, 1 cocktail, 250ml	10
Cocktails, strawberry daquiri, 1 cocktail, 250ml	8
Rum (40% alc.), 1 double shot (60ml)	7
Soda mix, flavoured vodka (4.8% alc.), 1 bottle (375ml)	11
Soda mix, rum and cola (5% alc.), 1 bottle (375ml)	12
Soda mix, whiskey and cola (5% alc.), 1 bottle (375ml)	11
Spirit mix, whiskey and dry ginger ale (5% alc.), 1 cocktail, 250ml	6
Vodka (40% alc.), 1 double shot (60ml)	6
Whiskey, 80 proof (40% alc.), 1 shot (30ml)	3
Whisky (40% alc.), 1 shot (30ml)	3
Wine, white or red, dry (12% alc.), small glass (120ml)	4

COFFEE, TEA AND FLAVOURED MILKS

Chocolate drink with full-fat milk, fast-food style, 300ml	15
Chocolate drink from chocolate powder with full-fat milk, 1 cup	8
Chocolate drink from chocolate powder with skim milk, 1 cup	5
Chocolate drink from chocolate powder with water, 1 cup	2
Chocolate drink, Hot Chocolate, sachet, 1 cup	4
Chocolate drink, MILO B-SMART with skim milk, 1 cup	7

Chocolate drink, MILO with reduced-fat milk, 3 tsp in 200ml	9
Chocolate drink, MILO with skim milk, 3 tsp in 200ml	7
Chocolate drink, NESQUIK with reduced-fat milk 3 tsp in 200ml	7
Chocolate drink, NESQUIK with skim milk, 3 tsp in 200ml	6
Chocolate drink with regular milk, caramel syrup and cream, 1 cup	11
Chocolate drink with soy milk, 1 cup	7
Coffee, NESCAFÉ CAFÉ MENU, cappuccino, skim, prepared, 150ml	2
Coffee, caramel macchiato with regular milk, 473ml	13
Coffee, chicory coffee powder, 1 tsp	1
Coffee, espresso, long black or instant, without milk, (1 cup)	0
Coffee, Turkish style, without milk, (1 cup)	3
Coffee, cappuccino or latte, with full fat milk (1 small,cup)	4
Coffee, cappuccino or latte, with full fat milk (1 medium cup)	5
Coffee, cappuccino or latte, with full fat milk (1 large cup)	7
Coffee, cappuccino or latte, with skim milk (1 small cup)	3
Coffee, cappuccino or latte, with skim milk (1 large cup)	4
Coffee, cappuccino or latte, with soy milk, (1 small cup)	4
Coffee, instant, with 2 tbsp (40mL) low fat milk, (1 cup)	1
Coffee, instant, with 2 tbsp (40mL) full fat milk, (1 cup)	2
Coffee, instant, with dash (20mL) full fat milk, (1 cup)	1
Coffee, instant, with dash (20mL) low fat milk, (1 cup)	0
Coffee, mocha or mochaccino with full fat milk, (1 cup)	6
Coffee, mocha or mochaccino with skim milk, (1 cup)	4
Frappuccino, coffee, 473ml	11
Frappuccino, light mocha, 473ml	7
Frappuccino, mocha with whipped cream, 473ml	16
Frappuccino, strawberries and cream with whipped cream, 473ml	21
Malted Milk, NESTLÉ, with skim milk, 1 glass	7
Milk, flavoured, fresh, chocolate or coffee, 600ml	20
Milkshake, café style, chocolate flavoured, reduced-fat milk, 1 cup	8
Milkshake, café style, chocolate flavoured, reduced-fat milk, no ice cream, 1 cup	7
Milkshake, café style, chocolate flavoured regular milk, no ice cream, 1 cup	10
Tea, chai latte with regular milk, 300ml	12
Tea, chai latte with skim milk, 342ml	9
Tea, Iced Tea, NESTEA, 500ml	6
Tea, regular or herbal, brewed from leaf or teabags without milk, 1 cup	0
Thickshake, fast-food style, made with reduced-fat milk, 1 cup	8

ENERGY, SPORTS AND BREAKFAST DRINKS

Caffeinated energy drink, 1 cup	6
Electrolyte sports drink, 600ml	8
High-protein breakfast drink, chocolate, 1 cup	14
Soy, chocolate, liquid breakfast, 350ml	14

JUICE AND CORDIAL

Coconut, fresh, mature, water or juice, 1 cup	3
Cordial base, 25% fruit juice, intense sweetened, 1 tbsp	0
Cordial base, less than 25% fruit juice, 1 tbsp	2
Cordial, diet lime, prepared as directed, 200ml	0
Cordial, undiluted, blackcurrant juice, concentrated, 2 tbsp	3
Drink, fruit flavoured, dry base, 1 tbsp	3
Drink, fruit flavoured, dry base, reduced sugar, 1 tbsp	3
Fruit drink, cranberry juice, intense sweetened, 1 cup	1
Fruit puree drink, apple and pear, ½ cup	5
Grenadine syrup, 3 tsp (15ml)	2
Juice, apple concentrate, 1 tbsp	1
Juice, apple or orange, ¾ cup (200ml)	4
Juice, breakfast style (orange, apple, pineapple and passionfruit), 1 cup	4
Juice, carrot, 1 cup	3
Juice, cranberry, 1 cup	5
Juice, fruit and vegetable, mixed, 1 cup	5
Juice, grape, 1 cup	7
Juice, lime, 1 cup	3
Juice, mango, ¾ cup (200ml)	4
Juice, pear, 1 cup	6
Juice, pomegranate, ¾ cup (200ml)	5
Juice, prune, 1 cup	6
Juice, tomato, salted, 1 cup	2
Juice, wild berry, 650ml	13

SMOOTHIES

Smoothie, low fat, mango, 1 cup	8
Smoothie, regular, mango, 1 cup	14

SOFT DRINKS

Cola, 375ml	8
Fruit flavour, 1 cup	4
Ginger ale, 125ml	2
Ginger beer, 375ml	8
Lemonade, 1 cup	4
Slurpee, cola flavoured, 185ml	3
Soft drink, average, 1 cup	3
Soft drink, average, intense sweetened, 1 cup	0
Tea, iced, 1 cup, commercial	5
Tea, iced, homemade, 1 cup	2
Tonic water, 375ml	6

WATERS

Glaceau, vitamin water, average all flavours, 500ml	5
Mineral water, flavoured, sweetened, average, 1 cup	3
Mineral water, natural, unsweetened, 1 cup	0
Water, carbonated or soda, 1 bottle	0

Eggs, fats, oils and cream

This section includes eggs prepared in a variety of ways, and fats, oils and creams including avocado, butter, margarine, and dairy and coconut cream.

EGGS (CHICKEN)

Egg, whole, poached or boiled, 1 jumbo egg (67g)	5
Egg, scrambled, cooked with fat, 1 egg (50g)	4
Egg, scrambled, cooked without fat, 1 egg (50g)	3
Egg, scrambled with 1 tbsp skim milk, 1 egg (53g)	4
Egg, whole, poached or boiled, 1 egg (47g)	3
Egg, whole, poached or boiled, 1 egg (53g)	4
Omelet cooked with fat, 1 cup (232g)	18
Omelet with cheese, cooked with fat, 1 cup (256g)	24

FATS, OILS AND CREAMS

Avocado, mashed, 1 tbsp (20g)	2
Butter or margarine, 1 tsp (5g)	2
Coconut, cream, 1 cup (255g)	23
Coconut, milk, reduced fat, canned, 1 cup (255g)	9
Coconut, milk, regular, canned, 1 cup (255g)	19
Cream, average, 1 tbsp (20g)	4
Cream, light (18% fat), 1 tbsp (20g)	2
Cream, reduced fat (25% fat), 1 tbsp (20g)	3
Cream, regular thickened (35% fat), 1 tbsp (20g)	3
Cream, regular thickened, light (~18% fat), 1 tbsp (20g)	2
Cream, rich or double thick (43% fat), 1 tbsp (20g)	4
Cream, whipped, 1 heaped tbsp (15g)	2
Cream, whipped, aerosol, reduced fat, ½ cup (31g)	3
Dairy blend butter and edible oil spread, 1 tbsp (19g)	7
Fat, solid, vegetable oil based, 1 tbsp (17g)	7
Garlic butter, 1 tbsp (20g)	7
Ghee, clarified butter, 1 tbsp (17g)	7
Lard, 1 tbsp (17g)	7
Margarine spread, 1 tbsp (20g)	7
Oil, any kind, 1 tbsp (18g)	8
Oil, any kind, 1 tsp (5g)	2
Oil, spray, 3-second spray (5g)	2
Polyunsaturated spread, reduced fat (40% fat), 1 tbsp (19g)	3

Fish and seafood

This section includes canned, cooked and raw fish and seafood.

CANNED SEAFOOD

Anchovy, canned in oil, drained, 1 small can of 12 fillets (49g)	4
Crabmeat, canned in brine, drained, 1 cup (145g)	4
Salmon, Australian, canned in brine, drained, 1 cup (210g)	16
Salmon, pink, canned in spring water, drained, 1 small can (95g)	4
Salmon, pink, canned in spring water, drained, 1 small can (105g)	6
Salmon, red, canned in brine, drained, 1 small can (105g)	9
Sardines, canned in water or tomato sauce, drained, ½ 90g can (45g)	4
Tuna, canned in oil, drained, 1 small can (80g)	8
Tuna, canned in water, drained, 1 medium can (185g)	7
Tuna, canned in water, drained, 1 small can (95g)	4
Tuna, flavoured, canned in oil, drained, 1 small can (80g)	7
Tuna, flavoured, canned in water, drained, 1 small can (80g)	4

COOKED SEAFOOD

Clam, boiled, 1 cup (158g)	8
Cod, smoked, steamed or poached, 1 fillet (100g)	5
Crab, various types, fresh only, boiled or steamed, pieces, 1 cup (125g)	4
Crab/seafood stick, 1 stick (67g)	5
Fish finger, grilled or baked, 1 finger (25g)	3
Fish, fillet, cooked in foil, microwaved or grilled, 1 fillet (100g)	5
Fish, fillet, crumbed, oven baked, 1 fillet (71g)	8
Flathead, crumbed/floured, fried in oil, 1 fillet (104g)	10
Lobster, steamed or boiled, 1 cup (153g)	7
Mussel, green, steamed or boiled, 1 cup (158g)	9
Oyster, baked or grilled, 1 oyster (12g)	1
Prawn, cooked, shelled, 12 large (88g)	3
Prawn, flesh only, cooked, 1 cup (158g)	6
Prawn, king (large size), baked or grilled, 1 prawn (16g)	1
Prawn, king (large size), fried in oil, 1 extra large (25g)	2
Salmon, fresh, grilled, 1 fillet (100g)	11
Salmon, smoked, sliced, 2 slices (30g)	2
Scallop, boiled, 1 cup (190g)	10
Scallop, fried, 1 scallop (16g)	1
Snapper, crumbed, fried in oil, 1 fillet (178g)	15
Squid or calamari, baked/grilled, 1 cup (95g)	4
Squid or calamari, crumbed, fried, 1 ring (22g)	3

RAW SEAFOOD

Fish paste or spread, 1 tbsp (20g)	1
Fish roe (caviar), black, 1 tbsp (19g)	1
Oysters, shelled, 12 oysters (120g)	4
Sushimi, salmon, Atlantic, 1 matchbox-size piece (30g)	3
Sushimi, tuna, yellowfin, 1 matchbox-size piece (30g)	1

Fruit

This section includes canned, stewed, dried and fresh fruit.

CANNED AND STEWED FRUIT

Apricot canned in pear juice, drained, 1 cup (220g)	4
Apricot canned in syrup, drained, 3 halves (50g)	1
Apricot canned in water, drained, ½ can (137g)	2
Cherries, sour, pitted, 5 cherries (30g)	4
Cherry, glacé/maraschino, ½ cup (102g)	13
Fruit salad canned in pear juice, drained, 1 cup (220g)	4
Fruit salad canned in syrup, drained, 1 cup (220g)	5
Fruit stewed with sugar, ½ cup (150g)	5
Fruit stewed without sugar, ½ cup (120g)	3
Lychee canned in pear juice, drained, 1 cup (252g)	9
Mixed fruit, peach and pear, canned in liquid, drained, ½ cup (125g)	4
Peach canned in syrup, drained, ½ peach (40g)	1
Peaches with liquid, ½ cup (125g)	4
Pear canned in pear juice, drained, 1 cup (240g),	5
Pear canned in syrup, drained, 1 cup (240g)	7
Pineapple canned in pineapple juice, drained pieces, 1 cup (200g)	3
Pineapple canned in water, drained, 1 slice (40g)	1
Prune stewed without sugar, 1 cup (167g)	4
Prune stewed with sugar, 1 cup (167g)	7
Rhubarb, stewed, 1 cup (254g)	2

DRIED FRUIT

Apple, dried, 8 rings (40g)	5
Apricot, dried, 5 medium halves or 3 whole (30g)	3
Berries, mixed (e.g., strawberry, raspberry, blueberry), dried, ¼ cup (38g)	4
Coconut, grated and desiccated, ¼ cup (19g)	6
Cranberry, dried, sweetened, ¼ cup (38g)	5
Currant, dried, ¼ cup (38g)	5
Date, dried, with stone, 3–4 medium (90g)	4
Fig, dried, 1 fig (19g)	1
Fruit leather, 1 strip (16g)	3
Mango, dried, 1 piece (5g)	1
Mixed fruit, dried, ¼ cup (44g)	6
Pawpaw (papaya) dried, sweetened, diced, ¼ cup (37g)	5

Pineapple, dried, sugar sweetened, 1 piece (28g)	4
Prune (dried plum), moist, pitted, 4 prunes (32g)	3
Sultanas, 1 tbsp (15g)	2
FRESH FRUIT	
Apple, 1 large (216g)	5
Apple, 1 medium (150g)	4
Apricot, 2 large (120g)	2
Banana, 1 large, 18cm (210g)	6
Banana, 1 medium (180g)	5
Banana, 1 small, 13cm (130g)	4
Banana, mashed, ½ cup (125g)	6
Blackberry, 10 berries (50g)	1
Blueberries, ½ cup (75g)	2
Boysenberry, 1 serve (39g)	1
Cherry, 16 medium (100g)	3
Coconut, fresh, mature fruit, flesh, 1 piece (45g)	6
Dates, 4 dates (160g)	3
Fig, unpeeled, 1 fig (50g)	1
Fruit salad, fresh, with melon, ½ cup (100g)	2
Fruit salad, fresh, deli style, ½ cup (120g)	6
Fruit salad, tropical, fresh, ½ cup (100g)	2
Grapefruit, ½ medium (100g)	1
Grapes, red globe, 1 small bunch (22 grapes) (118g)	4
Guava, 1 guava (90g)	1
Kiwifruit, 1 medium (100g)	2
Lychee, peeled, 1 lychee (10g)	0
Mandarin, peeled, 1 medium (86g)	2
Mango, peeled, 1 cheek (120g)	3
Mango, peeled, 1 medium (300g)	5
Mango, peeled, 1 small (174g)	4
Melon, honeydew, white skin, peeled, 1 slice (125g)	2
Melon, rockmelon, ½ small melon, flesh only (252g)	3
Melon, rockmelon, 1 cup (160g)	2
Melon, rockmelon, peeled, 1 slice (53g)	1
Mulberry, 1 cup (148g)	2
Nectarine, 1 large (151g)	3
Orange, 1 medium (230g)	4
Orange, 1 small (131g)	2
Passionfruit, 1 small (18g)	0
Pawpaw (papaya), 1 cup (148g)	2
Pawpaw (papaya), ½ medium (230g)	4

Peach, 1 large (145g)	3
Pear, brown skin, 1 medium (161g)	4
Pineapple, 1 slice (111g)	2
Plum, 2 medium (200g)	3
Pomegranate, 1 pomegranate (240g)	8
Rambutan, 1 fruit (16g)	1
Raspberry, fresh, 1 cup (140g)	3
Strawberry, 1 small punnet (250g)	3
Watermelon, 1 thick slice, ½ circle, 3cm (300g)	3
Watermelon, 1 thin slice, ½ circle, 1.5cm (150g)	2

Ice cream

TUBS OF ICE CREAM	
Original Classic Vanilla, (6% fat) PETERS, 1 scoop (46g)	4
Light 'n' Creamy, PETERS, 1 scoop (50g)	3
No Added Sugar, PETERS, calcium fortified, 2 scoops (94g)	4
Regular, full cream (10% fat), 1 scoop (50g)	5
Gelato, 1 scoop (50g)	3
ICE CREAM-RELATED PRODUCTS	
BILLABONG, 1 ice cream stick (70g)	4
Choc top, 1 ice cream (105g)	15
Lemonade ice confection, 1 bar (80g)	2
SKINNY COW, 1 stick (67g)	4
Soft-serve cone, small	7
Sorbet, 1 scoop (50g)	3
Sorbet, milk based, 1 scoop (50g)	5
Stick, chocolate coated, 1 stick (64g)	8
Stick, milk based, 1 stick (90g)	6
Sundae, fast-food style, 1 sundae (328g)	16
Super premium/rich ice cream, 1 scoop (50g)	9
Cone (empty), 1 cone	1
Waffle cone (empty), 1 cone	4
Syrup, chocolate, 1 tbsp (20g)	2
Syrup, chocolate, diet, 3 tbsp (60g)	1

Meat

This section includes both cooked and processed meats, such as ham, salami and corned beef, and poultry.

COOKED MEAT

Bacon, grilled, 1 rasher (34g)	5
Beef burger patty or rissole, grilled or fried without oil, 1 patty (75g)	7
Beef kebab, grilled or barbecued, 1 kebab (72g)	7
Beef, roast, deli style, 2 thin slices (86g)	7
Beef, silverside roast, untrimmed, baked or roasted, 1 slice (44g)	4
Beef steak, lean, rump or fillet, 1 medium (100g)	9
Beef steak, lean, T-bone, 1 medium (170g)	15
Beef, stewed, 1 cup (diced) (148g)	16
Beef, tail (ox tail), simmered, 1 cup (diced) (148g)	25
Frankfurt, canned, boiled, 1 cocktail size (10g)	1
Kangaroo steak, rump or loin fillet, grilled, 1 steak (65g)	5
Lamb cutlet, lean, grilled, 1 medium (100g)	10
Lamb rump, lean, grilled, 1 medium (100g)	11
Lamb kebab, grilled or barbecued, 1 kebab (72g)	9
Lamb loin chops, lean, grilled, 2 chops (120g)	13
Lamb roast, lean, 2 slices (85g)	8
Lamb stew or casserole, 1 cup (diced) (148g)	20
Pork, baked, 1 slice (28g)	2
Pork leg schnitzel, lean, dry-fried, 1 schnitzel (121g)	8
Pork loin chop, trimmed, grilled, 1 small (100g)	8
Pork spare ribs, lean and fat, grilled or barbecued, 1 rib (bone removed) (117g)	13
Pork stew or casserole, 1 cup (diced) (142g)	12
Saveloy, pork, battered, deep-fried, 1 frankfurt (51g)	8
Veal schnitzel steak, lean, crumbed and pan-fried, 1 small (120g)	13
Veal leg steak, lean, fried in oil, 1 steak (87g)	8
Veal leg steak, lean, grilled, 1 steak (87g)	7

PROCESSED MEAT

Beef, corned, canned, 1 slice (25g)	2
Beef, jerky, all flavours, 1 serve (28g)	4
Ham, lean (97% fat free), 4–5 thin slices (50g)	2
Ham, off the bone, trimmed, 2 large thick slices (100g)	5
Kabana or cabanossi, 1 piece (29g)	4
Meat paste or spread, 1 tbsp (19g)	2
Pastrami, 4 thin slices (80g)	4
Pâté, liverwurst, 1 tbsp (14g)	2
Prosciutto, 1 slice (20g)	2
Salami, 1 slice (23g)	5
Salami, peperoni, 1 slice (23g)	5
Salami, Polish, 1 slice (23g)	3
Sausage, cooked, small, 1 thick sausage, (70g)	9
Sausage, cooked, medium, 1 thick sausage (90g)	10
Sausage, cooked, medium, 1 thin sausage (60g)	6
Sausage, low fat (8%), cooked, 1 sausage (60g)	4
Sausage, reduced fat (15%), cooked, 1 sausage (60g)	5
Saveloy, pork, battered, deep-fried, 1 frankfurt (51g)	8
Spam, canned, 1 slice (20g)	3

POULTRY

Chicken breast fillet, grilled, lean and skinless, ½ large breast (86g)	7
Chicken thigh fillet, grilled, skinless, 1 medium (100g)	9
Chicken drumstick meat, roasted with skin, no bones, 1 large (125g)	13
Chicken drumstick and thigh, barbecued with skin and bones, 1 small (140g)	14
Chicken kebab, grilled or barbecued, 1 stick (72g)	5
Chicken kebab, satay, 1 stick (85g)	6
Chicken nuggets, 6 average (120g)	14
Chicken roll, processed luncheon meat, 1 slice (25g)	2
Chicken roll, processed luncheon meat, low or reduced fat, 1 slice (25g)	1
Chicken thigh, roasted, 1 small (110g)	9
Chicken, lean, stewed or braised, 1 piece (112g)	9
Chicken wings in Chinese honey marinade, 2 wings (100g)	8
Pâté de foie (chicken liver pâté), 1 tbsp (18g)	2
Quail, flesh and skin, baked, 1 quail (76g)	7
Turkey, roast, deli sliced, ready to eat, 1 slice (22g)	2

Nuts and seeds
This section includes both raw and roasted nuts and seeds.

NUTS AND SEEDS

Nut, almond, with skin, 10 nuts (12g)	3
Nut, Brazil, raw or blanched, 10 nuts (35g)	11
Nut, cashew, raw, 10 nuts (15g)	4
Nut, chestnut, roasted, 10 nuts (84g)	6
Nut, hazelnut, raw, 10 nuts (15g)	4
Nut, macadamia, raw, 10 nuts (20g)	7
Nut, macadamia, roasted with oil, 10 nuts (20g)	7
Nut and seed mix, 2 tbsp (20g)	6
Nut, peanut, with skin, raw, 10 nuts (8g)	2
Nut, peanut, without skin, roasted with oil, 10 nuts (8g)	3
Nut, pecan, 10 nuts (halved) (22g)	7
Nut, pine, raw, 1 tbsp (14g)	5
Nut, pistachio, 10 nuts (7g)	2
Nut, walnut, raw, 10 halves (15g)	5
Nuts, mixed (peanut, cashew, hazelnut, brazil nut), 10 nuts (14g)	4
Nuts, mixed (peanut, cashew, hazelnut, brazil nut), with dried fruit, ½ cup (76g)	19
Pumpkin seeds, hulled and dried, ¼ cup (37g)	10
Pumpkin seeds/pepitas, 1 tbsp (15g)	4
Seed, linseed or flaxseed, ¼ cup (44g)	10
Seed, linseed or flaxseed, LSA, 1 tbsp (12g)	3
Seed, poppy, 1 tbsp (12g)	3
Seed, sesame, 1 tbsp (11g)	3
Seed, sunflower, 1 tbsp (11g)	3

Rice, pasta and grains
This section covers pasta, rice, rice noodles and gnocchi, and grains including couscous, polenta, quinoa and semolina.

RICE, PASTA AND GRAINS

Couscous, cooked, 1 cup (157g)	8
Gnocchi, potato, cooked, ½ cup (70g)	8
Noodle, bean starch or cellophane, boiled, 1 cup (220g)	11
Noodle, rice, boiled, 1 cup (150g)	6
Noodle, wheat, Asian style, 1 cup (169g)	12
Noodles, plain, boiled, 1 cup (135g)	7
Pasta, non-wheat, boiled, 1 cup (126g)	7
Pasta, plain, boiled, ½ cup (75g)	5
Pasta salad with vegetables and bacon, 1 serve (129g)	9
Pasta salad with vegetables and cheese, 1 serve (45g)	3
Pasta salad with vegetables and mayonnaise, 1 serve (116g)	8
Pasta salad with vegetables, 1 serve (78g)	4
Pasta, salad, with vegetables, cheese and bacon, 1 serve (184g)	15
Pasta, white wheat flour with egg, boiled, 1 cup (195g)	13
Polenta, cooked in water without fat, ½ cup (98g)	7
Quinoa, cooked in water, 1 cup (195g)	10
Quinoa, cooked with milk, 1 cup (195g)	15
Rice, brown or white, boiled, ½ cup (80g)	5
Rice, wild, boiled, 1 cup (137g)	6
Semolina, prepared with milk, 1 cup (245g)	17
Semolina, prepared with water, 1 cup (245g)	13
Tapioca, pearl or seed style, boiled, 1 cup (265g)	5

Snacks, soups and takeaway foods
This section includes common snacks such as muesli bars, chips and popcorn, canned and dried soups, and takeaway meals including burgers, pizzas, curries, sushi, nachos and tacos, as well as deep-fried accompaniments like chips, dim sims, spring rolls and samosas.

SNACKS

Banana chips, ¼ cup (30g)	7
Breakfast bar, breakfast cereal, yoghurt or chocolate coated, 1 bar (25g)	5

Bar, breakfast or snack style, cereal and nut, 1 bar (40g) — 7

Bar, breakfast or snack style, cereal, plain or with dried fruit, 1 bar (22g) — 4

Bar, muesli, breakfast, fruit or snack style, 1 bar (30g) — 5

Bar, muesli, chocolate chip, 1 bar (31g) — 6

Bar, muesli, plain or with dried fruit, 1 bar (40g) — 7

Bar, muesli, wholegrain, 1 bar (20g) — 6

Bar, muesli, with added nuts, 1 bar (35g) — 7

Bar, rice cereal, chocolate and confectionery, LCM style, 1 bar (22g) — 4

Bar, rice cereal, with choc chip, LCM style, 1 bar (22g) — 5

Bar, sesame seed, 1 bar (45g) — 10

Bar, sesame seed, chocolate coated, 1 bar (45g) — 10

Chips, 20g pack — 6

Chips, 50g pack — 12

Chips, 100g pack — 24

Chips, 200g pack — 48

Hot chips, 1 small cup (150g) — 22

Plain corn chips, 1 medium packet (50g) — 12

Popcorn, 1 serve (100g) — 23

Popcorn, air popped, 2 cups (16g) — 3

Popcorn, cinema, with butter, 1 large container (115g) — 26

Pretzels, 10 pieces (60g) — 11

Wasabi peas, ¼ cup (30g) — 6

SOUPS

Asian style, with noodles, from dry mix, reconstituted with water, 1 cup (253g) — 4

Beef, broth style, condensed, canned, 1 cup (253g) — 5

Chicken, broth style, condensed, canned, 1 cup (253g) — 4

Cream of pumpkin with croutons, from dry mix, reconstituted with water (200ml) — 5

Cream variety, cup style, from dry mix, reconstituted with water, 1 cup (265g) — 5

Pea and ham soup, cup style, from dry mix, reconstituted with water, 1 cup (250ml) — 5

Minestrone, canned, 1 can (240g) — 5

Miso with radish, 1 cup (253g) — 2

Pumpkin, canned, 1 small bowl (300g) — 8

Vegetable, cup style, from dry mix, reconstituted with water, 1 cup (258g) — 3

Winter vegetable, 1 cup (250g) — 6

TAKEAWAY FOODS

Chicken burger with bacon, cheese, mayonnaise and lettuce, 1 burger (186g) — 18

Chicken burger with mayonnaise and lettuce, 1 burger (211g) — 20

Dim sim, meat and vegetable filling, deep-fried, 1 piece (50g) — 5

Dumpling, meat filled, Chinese style, steamed, 1 piece (97g) — 8

Dumpling, prawn filled, Chinese style, steamed, 1 piece (97g) — 6

Falafel, chickpea patty, fried, 2 small falafel (40g) — 5

Fish cake, deep-fried, 1 cake (80g) — 11

Fishburger with cheese, 1 burger (137g) — 16

Hamburger, 1 plain burger (beef patty with lettuce, tomato, onion and sauce) (246g) — 19

Hamburger, 1 with beef patty, fried egg and bacon, lettuce, onion and sauce (270g) — 29

Hamburger, 1 with beef patty, fried egg, lettuce, onion and sauce (266g) — 28

Hamburger, 1 with beef patty, onion, pickles and sauce (95g) — 11

Hamburger, 1 with 2 beef patties, cheese, onion, bacon and sauce (269g) — 34

Hamburger, 1 with 2 beef patties, cheese, salad, bacon and mayonnaise (233g) — 28

Nachos with beans, cheese and avocado, 1 serve (306g) — 41

Nachos with beef, beans, cheese and avocado, 1 serve (573g), — 60

Nachos with cheese, 1 serve (252g) — 34

Pizza, ham and pineapple, 1 slice (84g) — 10

Pizza, supreme, 1 slice (84g) — 9

Potato chips, deep-fried, salted, 1 small cup (150g) — 14

Potato wedges, 4 wedges (100g) — 6

Prawn curry, tandoori style, 1 prawn with sauce (23g) — 1

Samosa, vegetable, 1 piece (145g) — 18

Spring roll, deep-fried, 1 spring roll (64g) — 7

Sushi, California roll, 1 lunch box serve (260g) — 16

Sushi, chicken, 1 lunch box serve (260g) — 16

Sushi, meat (beef, pork, lamb), 1 lunch box serve (260g) — 16

Sushi, vegetarian, 1 lunch box serve (260g) — 16

Sushi, average, 3 small pieces (150g) — 7

Taco, 1 with beef, lettuce and sauce (219g) — 20

Taco, 1 with beef, lettuce, cheese and sauce (219g) — 23

Vegetables

This section includes starchy and non-starchy vegetables—fresh, canned or frozen—as well as legumes such as beans, peas and lentils. Note that unlike most non-starchy vegetables which have low counts and so are a bonus food, avocado is high in fat so will have higher counts.

STARCHY VEGETABLES

Cassava, baked without oil, 1 cup (diced) (139g)	13
Cassava, yellow flesh, peeled, raw, 1 cup (diced) (139g)	8
Creamed corn, ½ cup (125g)	4
Potato salad, 1 cup, homemade style (180g)	10
Potato salad, ½ cup deli-style (120g)	9
Potato, boiled, 1 large (220g)	9
Potato, boiled, 1 medium (150g)	6
Potato, boiled, 1 small (60g)	3
Potato, gems or nuggets, fresh or frozen, baked without oil, 10 pieces (88g)	3
Potato, gems, smiles, nuggets, fresh or frozen, fried in oil, 10 pieces (88g)	6
Potato in its jacket, 1 medium (150g)	5
Potato, mashed, with margarine and milk, ⅔ cup (150g)	8
Potato, mashed, reconstituted from dry powder with milk and butter, 1 cup (222g)	17
Potato, mashed, reconstituted from dry powder with milk and water, 1 cup (260g)	11
Potato, sweet, 2 pieces (200g)	6
Potato wedges, 3 large (75g)	8
Pumpkin, butternut, peeled, raw, 1 cup (120g)	3
Pumpkin, mashed, ½ cup (100g)	2
Pumpkin, wedge, 1 small piece (100g)	2
Sweetcorn, canned, drained, 1 cup (177g)	8
Sweetcorn, fresh on cob, boiled, drained, 1 ear (123g)	6
Sweetcorn, fresh on cob, large (200g)	9
Sweetcorn, fresh on cob, medium (100g)	5
Sweetcorn, fresh on cob, small (50g)	3
Sweetcorn, frozen, boiled, drained, 1 cup (173g)	8

NON-STARCHY VEGETABLES

Artichoke, globe, raw, 1 globe (133g)	1
Asparagus, raw, 3 spears (60g)	1
Avocado, ½ small (55g)	5
Avocado, ¼ medium (40g)	4
Avocado, mashed, 1 tbsp (20g)	2
Avocado, salad slice, 1 slice (13g)	1
Bamboo shoot, canned, drained, 1 cup (127g)	0
Beetroot, canned, drained, 1 slice (8g)	0
Beetroot, fresh, peeled, raw, 1 cup (grated) (144g)	3
Bok choy, 1 cup (chopped) (75g)	0
Broccoli, 1 cup (150g)	3
Brussels sprout, fresh, raw, 1 cup (93g)	1
Cabbage, red, raw, 1 cup (shredded) (95g)	1
Cabbage, white, raw, 1 cup (shredded) (86g)	1
Capsicum, green, raw, 1 cup (sliced) (85g)	1
Capsicum, red, raw, 1 cup (sliced) (85g)	1
Carrot, 1 medium carrot (140g)	3
Cauliflower, raw, 1 floret (13g)	0
Celery, raw, 1 stalk (14g)	0
Choko, peeled, raw, 1 choko (168g)	1
Cucumber, common, unpeeled, raw, 3 thin slices (26g)	0
Cucumber, Lebanese, unpeeled, raw, 3 thick slices (26g)	0
Dried vegetables, ¼ cup (40g)	2
Eggplant, raw, 1 cup (chopped) (87g)	1
Gherkin, pickled, drained, 1 gherkin (25g)	1
Ginger, 5 slices (11g)	0
Herbs, fresh, 1 tbsp (10g)	0
Kale, raw, 1 cup (chopped) (137g)	1
Leek, raw, 1 cup (sliced) (94g)	1
Lettuce, shredded, 1 cup (35g)	0
Mixed vegetables (parsnip and carrot), fresh, cooked and mashed, 1 cup (116g)	2
Mixed vegetables, frozen, boiled or microwaved, drained, 1 cup (142g)	3
Mushroom, common, raw, 1 cup (74g)	1
Mushroom, canned (in butter), ½ cup (100g)	2
Okra, boiled, drained, 1 cup (194g)	2
Olive, green or black, drained, 10 olives (40g)	4
Olive, green, pimento stuffed, drained, 10 olives (40g)	2
Onion, 1 medium onion (120g)	2
Onion, sautéed onion rings (in minimum oil), ½ cup (120g)	5
Onion, pickled, drained, 1 onion (30g)	1

Onion, spring, raw, 1 spring onion (15g)	0
Parsnip, peeled, raw, 1 cup (chopped) (125g)	3
Pea, green, fresh, raw, 1 cup (145g)	4
Radish, white skinned, peeled, raw, 1 radish (20g)	0
Salad, Caesar, with dressing, 1 cup (123g)	15
Salad, coleslaw, with dressing, 1 cup (200g)	11
Salad, Greek, with dressing, 1 serve (130g)	8
Sauerkraut, canned in brine, drained, 1 cup (150g)	1
Seaweed, nori, poached, 1 sheet (0.5g)	0
Shallot, peeled, raw, 2 bulbs (11g)	0
Snow pea, raw, 10 pods (33g)	0
Spinach, English, raw, 1 cup (chopped) (35g)	0
Spinach, baby, raw, 1 cup (35g)	0
Sprout, snow pea, raw, 1 cup (92g)	1
Squash, button, raw, 1 squash (40g)	0
Swede, peeled, raw, 1 cup (chopped) (140g)	1
Tomato, cherry, raw, 1 cherry tomato (17g)	0
Tomato, common, raw, 1 tomato (167g)	1
Tomato, semi-dried without oil, 1 piece (4.8g)	0
Tomato, sun-dried in vegetable oil, 1 piece (4.8g)	1
Tomato, sun-dried in vegetable oil, drained, 5 pieces (22g)	3
Tomato, whole, canned in tomato juice, 1 cup (250g)	2
Tomato, whole, canned in tomato juice, drained, 1 cup (185g)	2
Turnip, white, peeled, raw, 1 turnip (122g)	1
Zucchini, green skin, raw, 1 zucchini (101g)	1

BEANS, PEAS AND LENTILS

Bean, black, boiled, drained, 1 cup (211g)	10
Bean, green, fresh or boiled, drained, 1 cup (140g)	1
Bean, green, fresh, raw, 1 cup (120g)	1
Bean, cannellini, canned, drained, ½ cup (128g)	5
Bean, mixed, canned, drained, ½ cup (100g)	4
Bean salad, 3 bean mix, drained, 1 medium can (68g)	7
Bean salad, deli style, ½ cup (120g)	8
Beans, kidney, canned, drained, ½ cup (75g)	5
Beans, refried, canned, ½ cup (134g)	5
Chickpeas, canned, drained, ½ cup (75g)	5
Chickpeas, canned, drained, 1 small can (125g)	5
Lentils, canned, drained, ½ can (120g)	5
Tofu, marinated, Chinese honey, ½ packet (100g)	8
Tofu (soy bean curd), firm, 1 serve (100g)	3
Tofu (soy bean curd), silken or soft, 1 serve (100g)	2

Acknowledgements

Many heads are better than one, and for this book that was certainly true. Numerous people brought their knowledge, experience and ideas to create this book.

First of all, the young and passionate team of NESTLÉ and UNCLE TOBYS nutritionists, Nilani Sritharan, Anja Sussmann, Luke Gibson, Caitlin Hughes, Jutta Wright and Virginia Fazio, brought their knowledge and love of nutrition and food to the writing of the meals, snacks, treats and desserts, and drinks chapters.

Our chefs, Richard Brogan, Kristen McQueen and Belinda Farlow, created and tested recipes that will inspire you and show that nutritious eating can include beautiful food.

Our two wise women enabled the project: Katrina Koutoulas, NESTLÉ marketing manager, who is passionate about NESTLÉ and the company's journey to becoming the world's largest nutrition, health and wellness company; and Philippa Sandall, whose creative approach and years of publishing experience and wisdom led the team.

Finally, Sue Hines, her team from Allen & Unwin and our photographer Adrian Lander, understood our vision and have brought it to life in a beautiful book that I hope will inspire you to eat delicious food in a way that helps you achieve a happy weight and transform your life.

Bon appétit!

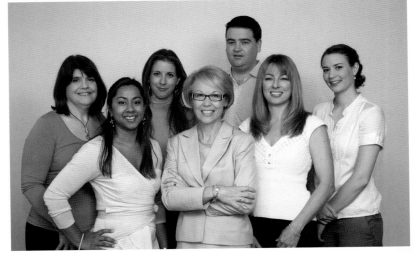

NESTLÉ and UNCLE TOBYS nutritionists, from left to right: Virginia Fazio; Nilani Sritharan; Anja Sussmann; Penny Small; Luke Gibson; Jutta Wright; and Caitlin Hughes. (May 2010)

Index

Recipe Index